Deaf and Hearing
Siblings in Conversation

Deaf and Hearing Siblings in Conversation

Marla C. Berkowitz *and*
Judith A. Jonas

Foreword by Martha A. Sheridan

McFarland & Company, Inc., Publishers
Jefferson, North Carolina

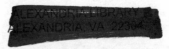

Library of Congress Cataloguing-in-Publication Data

Berkowitz, Marla C., 1964–
 Deaf and hearing siblings in conversation / Marla C.
Berkowitz and Judith A. Jonas ; foreword by Martha A.
Sheridan.
  p.   cm.
 Includes bibliographical references and index.

 ISBN 978-0-7864-7825-5 (softcover : acid free paper) ∞
 ISBN 978-1-4766-1513-4 (ebook)

 1. Deaf—Family relationships. 2. Deaf—Means of
communication. 3. Brothers and sisters of people with
disabilities. 4. Brothers and sisters—Psychological aspects.
I. Jonas, Judith A., 1943– II. Title.
 HV2380.B47 2014
 305.9'082—dc23   2014023703

British Library cataloguing data are available

Cover image © iStock/Thinkstock

Printed in the United States of America

McFarland & Company, Inc., Publishers
 Box 611, Jefferson, North Carolina 28640
  www.mcfarlandpub.com

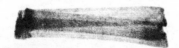

Acknowledgments

Each of us had a circle of people who have been there from the very beginning of the birth of our project many years ago. They've been bystanders but not without a significant purpose, whether they knew it or not. We are forever indebted for their confidence and trust in our journey.

To the siblings who let us do face-to-face interviews: Welcoming us to your homes, baring your sibling experiences without hesitation, and trusting us with your deepest thoughts is beyond gratitude. Without you this book would never have existed.

To the Lawrence W. Levine Foundation: We are extremely grateful for the extended financial support from Russell Kane, who had been a childhood friend of Marla's for more than forty years, for soliciting the funding on behalf of the foundation for the interviews, travel expenses, and other operational costs to complete the research study on sibling relationships.

To Dr. Brenda Brueggemann: You have been our ardent supporter and editor, boosting our confidence that studying deaf and hearing adult siblings was critical and timely. Your expertise in addressing the cohesiveness of our preliminary manuscript, complete with your warmth, wit and salient comments, steered us in the right direction.

From Marla Berkowitz:

To Charisse: Your love and encouragement never wavered, challenging me to write with clarity from our countless chats about my work on siblings.

To Hannah: Your everyday reminder to get up and take me out for our long walks is a lifesaver. You've been the most patient and understanding canine ever!

To Mom, Dad and Arnold: What you have provided for me is never taken for granted. Your love and devotion were plentiful, especially with teaching me the determination to navigate efficiently in this world.

To Julie and Joseph: With gratitude, your frankness in sharing incredible perspectives, which shed light on my understanding you slightly better. It gives me hope that in the days ahead we can conquer the hurdles of our distant sibling relations.

To Danny, Benjamin, Mia, Ayla, Sophie and Danielle: My dearest nephews and nieces, watching you grow up to be as loving as you are, reminds me that being a sibling is to be cherished.

To Rich, Lisa, and Michelle: Even though you came into my family later through our parents' marriage, I look forward to the days when I can get to know you and your children better.

To Judy: Our weekly and monthly sessions, and our years of work together remotely, were truly the best and most rewarding I've ever experienced in ways you've never imagined. Thank you for being such a great role model, for being a friend, for sharing openly about your life confirming the joys of being a sibling.

And ... to those who have seen me working on this project nonstop, I offer my deepest gratitude for your inquisitiveness, rooting, and years of patience!

From Judy Jonas:

To my husband, Peter: You're always there for me, supporting my many muses.

To my brother, Larry: We're simpatico. We've never had a fight.

To my sister, Mary Ann: Unknowingly, you led the way.

To my daughter, Deborah: You guided us through our tangle of data and listened.

To my daughter, Wendy: Your support and faith in my work were constant.

To Ed and Joan, Arnie and Nina: As lifelong friends, your encouragement was invaluable, recognizing this was a huge undertaking.

To JoAnn: You see, we're finally done.

To Eileen Forestal: You gently led me to the DEAF-WORLD.

To Marla Berkowitz, first my teacher, then a colleague, and now my friend who constantly challenged me to absorb and understand the depth and breadth of the DEAF-WORLD.

Table of Contents

Foreword

by Martha A. Sheridan

Most of us have drawn or painted family pictures and many of us have siblings who were depicted in these subjective works of art. No two paintings by siblings from a family will be the same because perception is in the eye of the beholder brought to view through the brushstrokes of our separate, yet connected minds and hearts. Rarely, if ever, do siblings have the chance to discuss their observations of these powerful reciprocal influences and outcomes and come to know each other and themselves through this personal reflection.

This book is not about just any ordinary relationship between brothers and sisters. Marla Berkowitz and Judy Jonas have begun an important and long overdue conversation about deaf and hearing sibling relations where we would assume that opportunities for shared communication and meanings are complicated by the lack of a common language or an imbalance in communication access. Relationship dynamics in families with deaf and hearing siblings have remained a mystery as researchers have historically focused their energies on the experiences of deaf children and those of their parents. Yet a whole image is made up of the sum of its parts, and to more fully understand the experiences and constructions of deaf-member families, we need to paint a complete landscape, including every part of the whole.

Co-researchers Marla Berkowitz, who is deaf with hearing siblings, and Judy Jonas, who is hearing with one deaf and one hearing sibling, have taken steps to complete this picture through phenomenological interviews with twenty-two deaf and hearing siblings. Inspired by their own personal experiences, the authors take us on an intimate and very personal journey through the lives and experiences of deaf and hearing siblings. The authors supplemented the narratives provided by their research participants with creative

1

stories to highlight and give context to their findings. The stories shared by their study participants are sometimes joyful, sometimes painful, yet always insightful. Readers who are themselves members of deaf-hearing sibling dyads will see themselves mirrored in these powerful and deeply personal narratives. As a deaf person, in a family with deaf and hearing siblings, I felt a strong kinship with the storytellers in this book as I reflected on my own similar family encounters.

This is a groundbreaking work complementing the seminal qualitative work of Paul Preston's *Mother, Father, Deaf* (1994), about the experiences of hearing children of deaf parents, Meadow-Orlans, Mertens, and Sass-Lehrer's *Parents and Their Deaf Children: The Early Years* (2002), a work about the experiences of parents of deaf children from birth through early elementary school, and my own *Inner Lives of Deaf Children: Interviews and Analysis* (2001) and *Deaf Adolescents: Inner Lives and Lifeworld Development* (2008), which are phenomenological explorations of the perceptions of deaf children and adolescents into their developmental lifeworlds. Together, these and other works (e.g. Spencer, Erting and Marschark, 2000) are contributing to a fuller, more holistic understanding of the individual and family contexts and experiences of deaf-member families.

Students in education, social work, psychology, counseling, interpreting, deaf studies, audiology, family studies, infant and toddler programs and health care professions will all appreciate, enjoy, and learn from the stories and insights shared in this book. They will be inspired and equipped to bring a fresh approach to their professional relationships. On a more personal level, parents, deaf adults, grandparents, adult siblings and extended family members will find the book especially enlightening as they seek to know and understand themselves and their unique family paintings. Discussion questions at the end of the book aid us in continuing the conversations that Berkowitz and Jonas begin.

This pioneering work allows us to see beyond the surface of a painted canvas. It takes us into the depths of the multiple meanings of the participants' renditions of deaf-hearing sibling relations and, consequently, enhances our understanding of entire family systems.

Dr. Martha Sheridan is a professor of social work at Gallaudet University and the author of two texts: *Inner Lives of Deaf Children: Interviews and Analysis* (2001) and *Deaf Adolescents: Inner Lives and Lifeworld Development* (2008).

Preface

"The sibling relationship is perhaps the most long-lasting and most influential relationship of a person's life."
                    —Powell & Gallagher 1993, xiii.

Are you close with your sibling? Is s/he deaf or hearing? Does s/he sign? Why or why not?

Numerous conversations of this sort among ourselves and people we knew compelled us to research the intensities of relationships between deaf and hearing adult siblings. We've also aimed to identify the tools these siblings used to either nurture or obstruct opportunities for fostering healthy relationships. Intensities of sibling relationships from best friends to enemies led us to ask this question: How well do you know your sibling? We began by looking at ourselves. We were each raised by hearing parents who did not sign. Marla Berkowitz has a distant relationship with her siblings, whereas Judy Jonas has had, as an adult, a close, loving relationship with hers. We've created a balanced text—aware of our own baggage while staying as neutral as possible—and respecting the sibling experiences of the deaf and hearing adults we interviewed.

Siblings generally outlive their parents; when they're gone, siblings are the ties that are left. Why not cherish these people who know us longer than anyone else? This book looks at deaf and hearing adult sibling relationships within the historical context of the nineteenth to twenty-first centuries after the Conference of Milan 1880 banned sign from deaf schools, an event affecting families with deaf and hearing members for over a hundred years. The isolation resulting from the Milan edict has a made lasting impression on deaf and hearing siblings. This pilot study entailed interviews with ten families of deaf and hearing adult siblings ranging from ages of twenty-two to seventy-eight years old. Based on the interviews, we've identified the perspectives of deaf and hearing siblings describing how they interact with their sibling. Pseudonyms are used to protect the privacy of the interviewees.

A Hassidic proverb—"Tell someone a fact and you reach their minds; give them a story and you touch their souls"—led us to create a collection of fictionalized stories, stemming from authentic events as told to us in these siblings' lives. Based on work developed by other researchers, we have identified significant interactions between deaf and hearing siblings and how these might define their relationship on a continuum ranging from intimate to hostile (Cicirelli 1995, Gold 1989). Twenty-two siblings is a small sample of subjects, the siblings we interviewed represented almost every degree of closeness on the continuum. Although family members make up the entire family functioning within the home, our text does not include parental perspectives, though through our siblings' interviews, the parents' actions were disclosed. Their decisions reflected the framework and early patterns of how family members—deaf and hearing—communicate with one another. For some family members, the precedent was set, remaining throughout their adult lives. For others, it was a springboard, triggering opportunities for change in how siblings can interact with one another.

As researchers, we are extremely attuned towards how other researchers study deaf people or people with a disability. When we explored the literature of siblings and family systems in a variety of contexts, earlier research on families with disabled children tended to focus on how the child with a disability affected the "normal" child but neglected to address how the person with a "disability" responded to their "normal" family. For us, then, the relationship dynamics seem oddly unidirectional. In addition, the majority of research regarding deaf and hearing siblings focused on children. We take interest in discussing general societal attitudes toward people with disabilities, and naturally, we have a personal interest in deaf people. Our common thread throughout the text is the impact of how stigma hovered over the lives of deaf and hearing siblings. Our work confronts these issues directly for the first time by our very presence: deaf and hearing adult sibling insiders who separately have gained access to the thoughts and experiences of deaf and hearing adult siblings, using qualitative methods and phenomenological interviews. Using a snowballing technique to locate deaf adults with hearing siblings, our intention was not to seek out these siblings with distinct identities within the deaf community, such as those who use Cued Speech and later signed, or those who use cochlear implants and never learned to sign. However, in our study, we uncovered additional variables: deaf-blind siblings, and deaf families with the sibling as the only hearing person. By the nature of their uniqueness, we did not specifically address their ramifications except in the context of how these siblings interacted with one another. Each of these, along with deaf siblings with deaf parents, could be studied to determine the specific dynamics of those sibling relationships.

Other areas of scholarship pertaining to families with deaf and hearing members deserve study. We tapped the areas of "isms" (audism, racism, sexism, etc.) and discussed how they contributed to sibling relationships, yet there are limitations to this pioneering work. The focus of this scholarship was to identify and show the depth of closeness in deaf and hearing adult siblings, including how the cultures they encountered might have contributed to the type of relationship they have with one another.

In family systems literature, optimal healthy family functioning has always been the ideal goal, consisting of multidirectional interactions among family members. Based on the fact that ninety percent of deaf children have hearing parents, it is imperative to look at the language used at home among parents and siblings as well as at school, in the neighborhood and in the larger community. We have identified a variety of communication systems among the siblings we interviewed affecting not only their interactions but consequently the relationship itself. In addition, we found cultural assumptions, unique to either the deaf or hearing experiences, that led to sibling conflicts. Interestingly, we also have identified tools they used to address these issues, which brought them closer to one another.

This book is divided into three sections using a narrative approach. The first section, "Emergence of a Sibling," begins by describing our work as a deaf-hearing team, as well as how our experiences as deaf and hearing siblings gave birth to this text. "Milan Impact" details how the historical realities stemming from changes in deaf education with respect to language, culture and communication modalities, permanently dominated siblings' lives. The final section, "Sibling Buddies," portrays how deaf-hearing sibling relationships are constantly evolving. Each interaction attempts to balance their worldview, for those who are committed to the belief that their sibling is a lifelong friend. Family harmony is achieved by not only acknowledging but *acting* on the belief that whatever affects one family member affects all members.

Affirming our sisters and brothers is like a stamp of self-approval.
—Marla C. Berkowitz and Judith A. Jonas

Introduction

As most genealogists would say, studying your family history begins with you. Knowing where you come from or about your grandparents or parents and their siblings' names, birth and death dates give us a reference for belongingness. Out of curiosity, many of us search for details about family members rather than merely accepting the facts of our ancestry. We are that inquisitive, striving to get the unusual, interesting tidbits about our family members' attributes and why they did what they did. Similar physical and personality traits of our ancestors either amuse or annoy us. By asking questions or engaging in conversations about events in our lives with family members or unrelated individuals, we often discover there are different perceptions to a memory that happened so long ago. Yet we are baffled at the question: Is it worth rehashing the past? For some of us the truth prevails, while for others, moving forward unknowingly may be the safest way. However, family is still everything to us, whether we readily admit it or not.

When we choose to talk about our siblings, we do it out of a sense of purpose: they have been and continue to be part of our lives. Sharing stories about them also confirms we are ready to reveal a deeper intimacy to our spouses, children, friends, acquaintances or service providers for how it defines us as a sibling in our family. Daily conversations about our families may be a common topic for discussion, but for some people it enters unchartered territory they would rather not talk about. Still there exists an untapped feeling inside of us which often cannot be explained—unless you are a sibling. Being a sibling is an emotional attachment that has grown on us, marking it as an experience that will always be part of us. Whether it is a birth of a sibling, adoption or a foster sibling, the sibling relationship is derived from hourly, daily, weekly, monthly, and accumulated years, of interactions. Building relationships is complex, especially when all we have is words, gestures and non-verbal forms of communication to create them in the first place. As time passes, our interactions come to form habitual ways that may or may not foster trust, respect and admiration for one another as a sibling. Ultimately however, we expect our siblings to know us as well as we think we know them.

Often when people ask if we are close with our siblings, it is their way of assessing the degree of intimacy in our lives. When this occurs, the boundaries expand from being private about ourselves to sharing personal information about ourselves to people we meet, always checking whether it's safe. Some siblings share stories about their siblings as a means of seeking mutual understanding, even including their harmless bickering. Others describe how they and their siblings share a common enemy, creating a co-dependency; there is a survivor's need in their sibling bond. And there are siblings who describe their closeness as middling or so-so, not close, but not distant either. Some define sibling closeness by creating an overall synthesized experience, interpreted or possibly misinterpreted into a single story. In contrast, our approach is to emphasize that sibling relationships are fluid and ever evolving throughout our lives. By looking at a continuum of intensities of sibling closeness ranging from intimate to hostile, it can be a way to take a step back and reassess our feelings about our sibling (Cicirelli 1995, Gold 1989). This analysis may lead us to jump start an interaction with our siblings. For some siblings, the relationship may have taken a turn for the worse, resulting in a complete halt, while for others, connecting or reconnecting to a sibling is seen as a worthwhile pursuit, depending on changing circumstances.

The single events as told to us by the people we interviewed portray multiple angles using different genres: one person's narrative, fictionalized conversations based on the actual events in siblings' lives, and anecdotal vignettes directly from the interviews. The genres were written to make it accessible to the multiple levels of linguistic and academic skills among prospective readers. Stories were specifically designed as an "easy read" to clearly identify the challenges enmeshed in sibling relationships and to give readers the opportunity to see that they are not alone—that other siblings have similar experiences. Simultaneously, we created a balance honoring the differing perspectives of siblings who live as deaf and hearing individuals. While it may appear that hearing status is the defining attribute, instead we've identified subtle distinctions emerging in the behavior of siblings surrounding how they adapt to one another, either inhibiting or nurturing sibling bonds. During the process of analyzing the sibling relationships between deaf and hearing adults, as researchers we present the deaf perspective, rarely seen or heard in many scholarly studies about sibling relations. For decades, traditional studies published the hearing perspectives. Deaf and hearing perspectives are not oppositional perspectives; instead they are simply the perspectives of how the person encountered the experience.

As authors our objective was to acknowledge the deaf and hearing experience while simultaneously presenting alternative possibilities that these experiences, by their very nature, are also in the context of being siblings. That the deaf perspective we know today comes from being marginalized daily in their interactions with hearing people is not a new phenomenon. Yet, deaf siblings confront their isolation with resiliency, evolving from daily encounters with people who do not sign in the family, the workplace, and their communities. Often the deaf perspective is misunderstood as being "emotionally immature" either by expressing their anger, possibly through yelling, behaving disruptively, or not caring when their authentic bluntness to the family and sibling experience is merely a response to the disempowerment they feel surrounded by loved ones. Their hearing counterparts' responses are scrambled with witnessing the injustice, feelings of helplessness and confusion.

Our readers will also see how an influential man, who was well connected in many circles, was sought as a respected leader at the 1880 Conference of Milan. Using his deaf wife as a model example, this led the educators all over the world to enforce a communication policy in deaf education: forbidding sign and requiring speech and lipreading only. The beliefs, policies and training of educators and medical practitioners stemming from Milan have successfully been established as the mainstream objective. Even though the Milan Conference is ancient history, the goal to find a cure for deafness is not without tensions from many who have pleaded, not only for recognition as a cultural, linguistic group, but who seek authenticity within themselves and from others as human beings. Social justice activists tried to counter the consequences of the Milan edict, but they were up against centuries of forced marginalization towards people who are deaf. Deaf and hearing family members were the carriers of a stigma, the deaf attribution, in every aspect of their lives.

Access to mainstream society is a stepping stone to economic, political, and social opportunities. By digging deeper and identifying how the stigma is enmeshed in attitudes and behaviors acquired and held onto by previous generations as well as current society, deaf and hearing siblings have long-term opportunities to improve their interactions and relationship. Siblings acquire ways of interacting from parental and educators' modeling. Then what fosters family harmony? We've identified the communication patterns of human interactions. Do they tend to interrupt when others are talking? Do they maintain eye contact? Do they sit down and talk during meal times, paying attention when everyone has a chance to tell about their day? Do they turn away while others are still talking to them? These questions focus on communication patterns, but clear and distinct behaviors have emerged with deaf and hearing siblings, based on auditory and visual cues. Our analysis addresses the tensions surrounding these issues, regardless of the degrees of sibling closeness.

Writing about siblings is revealing hidden family secrets. When we began our work as researchers, the interview process was almost like having a conversation with a therapist in our head. Sibling stories have rocked us, pushed our buttons, and brought out the worst or best in us. Selfishly, by learning how other deaf and hearing siblings in different stages of their lives responded to their daily stresses, it gave us insights to ponder in our own lives. It brought clarity, even joy and despair, yet at the same time the need for healing was a necessity for our emotional well-being. Even if we have yet to resolve our own sibling tensions, the pathway widened opportunities for responding to the interactions with our sisters and brothers in healthier ways. By comparing our sibling relationships with those of siblings we met, it gave us a framework: the search for a common ground to bond.

As authors, we begin the text as siblings, highlighting our backgrounds, our personal and professional experiences and how we live our lives as siblings. Unlike colleagues who know each other well collaborating in their respective offices, we were mere acquaintances. The conditions for partnership was each had to have a sibling who was either deaf or hearing, be fluent in American Sign Language (ASL) to communicate with one another, and be a social justice activist. How did two people, three states apart, write a book together, where we needed to blend our ideas, every phrase and every word? Interactive conversations were essential, not only for our role as authors, but in our commitment to keeping the perspectives of the siblings we interviewed. Our process became the defining challenge, especially since our sibling experiences were at opposite ends of closeness. Never anticipating how our intense and intimate conversations would bare our innermost vulnerabilities, we never wavered.

Early in our writing journey we had lengthy discussions and engaged in research about whether to use the upper case or the lower case letter D when we used the word deaf in our text. For close to thirty years, it had been common for authors to highlight the big D or little d, whether in their scholarly texts or lay articles, often with lengthy footnoted explanations, for the purpose of defending the existence of a cultural-linguistic deaf group. However, we've read that scholars and lay authors were inconsistent in their usages of the lower- and upper-case word, and have begun to question the purposes served by these distinctions (Brueggemann 2009). In addition, since the deaf community is diverse with multiple identities, our work is specifically geared at those who self-identify themselves as part of the DEAF-WORLD.[1] Since our focus on being a sibling transcended our need to single out any distinct trait of anyone's group affiliation, the particularity surrounding the lower case or upper case became moot. The DEAF-WORLD we describe is not a separate entity in society, but an existence of a group with its own language, culture and people co-existing in the mainstream. Those who are part of the DEAF-WORLD describe themselves as proponents of ASL and have had formative experiences in a deaf environment with native and near-native signers. Other communities, such as the Amish, feminists, or even groups who share a common interest with their own jargon, such as techs in Silicon Valley, share similar attributes that distinguish themselves from outsiders.

The DEAF-WORLD exists within the deaf community, which may be somewhat confusing to outsiders. When describing the deaf community, depending on whom you talk with or the context being discussed, it is often based on the identities of people gathered in specific places such as deaf clubs, silent dinners or retreats, deaf nights out, national, state and local conferences, deaf exhibitions, or other deaf events. How do hearing sisters and brothers of deaf siblings identify themselves to one another or when they are in the DEAF-WORLD? Being hearing has a double meaning: Born hearing is a biological definition, but H. Dirksen Bauman defines hearing identity as a "social construction" and "a profoundly different way of being in the world." When a ten-year-old deaf boy at a school for the deaf told Bauman, "You are hearing," for the first time Bauman awakened to the experience of being in the DEAF-WORLD, an "epistemological and cultural border that separates the Deaf and hearing worlds" (Bauman, *Open Your Eyes: Deaf Studies Talking*, 2008, viii). Many of the siblings we interviewed had similar experiences in which another identity, "becoming Hearing," was revealed, like the layers of an onion. Some realized they had no choice but to be, or might want to be, part of their sibling's DEAF-WORLD.

Another item throughout the text deserved a closer look: Sign. In the DEAF-WORLD, the definition for several lexical items have no equivalents in English. The term American Sign Language, conveyed in signed form, is ASL and capitalized in print to state its legitimacy as the official language used by native and near-native users. However, English uses the word "sign" in many different forms following English grammar rules. As a consequence, we've chosen to use the word "Sign," not ASL, referring to forms of signing following English word order. However, in the DEAF-WORLD, ASL has two discrete vocabulary terms: one sign states the person is fluent in ASL; the other sign refers to person who uses another form of signing, either as "learning how to sign" or "not skilled," or "lacks non-grammatical ASL features." In English, the word *sign* does not show these distinctions. For these reasons, when the interviewees were ambiguous about whether they were referring either to ASL or another form of signing, we use the lower-case "s" in the word sign.

From the interviews we had, in spite of the variety of communication modalities, siblings' objective was to understand and be understood. Our work is the platform for siblings who are deaf and hearing to begin having conversations. It is the place for siblings to analyze and understand how monitoring, facilitation or interpreting dictates the behaviors of both deaf and hearing siblings at family events, as they form partnerships with deaf and hearing family members. This text also presents the complexity surrounding using ASL interpreters at family events: The presence of a third party forces a shift in intimacy, changing the dynamics that often leaves deaf and hearing siblings feeling uneasy. However, rather than perpetuating the isolation among deaf and hearing siblings, the opportunities to get to know one another become available.

Professionals who work with deaf and hearing families are the closest in recognizing the severity of isolation and its impact on deaf and hearing siblings, yet there are many gaps in providing solutions. When families seek guidance from professionals, they are often sidetracked into single-focused positions on language approaches and educational issues, leaving them more bewildered and frustrated than ever. Early parental decisions affect every aspect of the deaf child's education, interpersonal and social skills, and overall well-being. Hearing siblings are witnesses and live with the lasting effects woven into their lives. For some, the sibling relationship becomes the final product molded by the lack of resources and tools either unavailable or ineffectively applied. However, for other siblings, by virtue of their differences, they've found ways to nurture their bonds. They turn to one another, believing "the life of anyone with a sibling begins with a sidekick and traveling companion who can be with you the entire way. Wasting that relationship is folly of the first order. It's true when we're kids, it's true when we're adults, and it's surely true when we're aging and alone" (Kluger, *The New Science of Siblings*, 2006, 290).

Another factor contributing to the dilemma of fragile sibling relationships is the kind of help families receive. In the last decade or two, deaf professionals have been trained as social workers, psychologists, therapists, guidance counselors, audiologists, case managers, rehabilitation counselors, and physicians. Why are many of them not sought for their professional expertise? Does a pervading stigma remain ingrained in the psyches of those who fear interacting with deaf professionals? Is it because they sometimes do not share the same language and have had different life experiences? Or are employers unwilling to invest in deaf professionals, preventing them from providing services to families in the first place? Even though communication is key to any relationship, our interviews with deaf and hearing siblings led us to new insights and laid the groundwork for understanding how they address the inevitable tensions surrounding their interactions.

This book presents an overarching overview of how interacting with a deaf family member reflects the larger society's attitudes and beliefs that have pervaded families' lives. They may appear to be isolated issues, but they are a microcosm of the mainstream. These efforts require a shift in how we interact with one another daily, either in person or through social media, especially toward people who are not like us. This text is a pioneering work; little has been written about this topic. For the first time, we aim to expose layers of sibling interactions that others have not addressed, made possible by the stories siblings told us during lengthy free-formed, unstructured interviews. Their stories introduce a change in world view—using the lens of deaf and hearing siblings—to achieve family harmony.

PART ONE

THE EMERGENCE OF A SIBLING

Solo Dining While Growing Up

When my whole family sat down at the dinner table
There was always
a lot to eat from corner to corner

There was always conversation
between forks and spoons

There was always conversation
between glasses and cups

There was always conversation
between napkins

There were always
empty plates and empty bowls

But the knife that laid between them all—
from mouth to ear—
from mouth to eye—

cut me off.

By Curtis Robbins (Robbins 2002)

1

How Conversations Began

"Being different, so you 'stand out' is a positive thing about having a deaf brother."—Newman

Family conversations are so personal. Intimately involved in our sibling experiences, we strive to know more about each other, projecting our humanity towards one another. A flood of shared memories, emotions, or thoughts eliminate the need for explanations—resulting in unspoken and presumed understandings. Conversation among family members is the essence of intimacy. The diner in the poem was not alone, yet he was. At his table, multiple conversations happened simultaneously. Did anyone notice that Curtis's plates and bowls were empty? He didn't crave the salads, soups or desserts. Silently, he spent a lifetime using his eyes—chasing his family's conversations.

Looking back to the year 2002 when we met in Manhattan, as potential authors, we instantly shared our sibling experiences as well as those of deaf and hearing siblings we knew. Our conversations led to a full-blown research project. Through personal or public recruitment efforts, we contacted twenty-six families. The twenty-two individuals, from ten families, came to us through a snowballing technique, first identifying deaf siblings, then following up with their hearing siblings. Separately, Marla interviewed ten deaf adults; Judy interviewed twelve of their hearing siblings. The youngest sibling was 22, the oldest 78, with every decade in between represented. Since we used face to face, in-depth interviews as opposed to structured questionnaires, we uncovered their sibling relationship's nuances, validated mutual shared experiences and shed light on the tools used to create a range of feelings from harmony to hostility between siblings.

Although we had the same set of questions prepared, our preference was to search for stories that left a mark, stories that recounted the most memorable sibling experiences throughout their life's passages. During the initial part of each interview, we provided a brief description of the project, asked our interviewees to sign a release giving us permission to conduct the interview, and assured confidentiality. Preserving confidentiality was two-pronged: within the DEAF-WORLD, and within any given family with a deaf member. Since the DEAF-WORLD is a place where associations make it easy to identify someone in the community comprised of many self-acclaimed identities, we scrupulously avoided the risk of exposing identities by not including any siblings' education history and current occupation. Equally important, we used siblings' phrases and perspectives to represent a group of siblings with a common trait and portrayed how their siblings responded without attributing a comment to any specific sibling.

We have made ourselves the exception. Our intention is to clearly distinguish ourselves as authors, but we too are siblings, and our siblings are part of who we are. It was not feasible to even imagine our journeys without including their thoughts, whether in comparison to ours or of other siblings. By virtue of their personalities, their wisdom, and strength, our sibling peers have shaped our perceptions, attitudes, and feelings, and have challenged us in every way possible. They have taught us the significance of having a sibling relationship as opposed to not having one. Without them, this book would not exist. The truth is even more convincing: our siblings are embedded into our well-being, as individuals, whether toxic, as our best friends, or anything in between. They have been and continue to be a part of our lives.

In our conversation, *which was the interview process,* we sought and collected standard information about the sibling's personal background: number of siblings in the family, ages, educational achievement, and the type of communication used with family members as children and as adults. We value this information to help us understand the historical context of the decade in which each was raised. For example, growing up in the 1940s as opposed to the 1970s shed light on society's perceptions of people who are different with respect to placing them in institutions or living at home with their families. The interviews ranged from one and a half hours to as long as three hours. Interestingly, most of these siblings had never had a lengthy talk with anyone about their experiences of being a sibling.

Both of us began the interviews by asking this general open-ended question: "Tell me about your positive and negative experiences growing up with a sibling." With encouragement, we wanted their stories to help us identify where they are in their relationship with their sibling; in turn, we shared some of our own experiences. We used specific follow-up questions to stimulate further conversation about: communication; how they identified themselves; family dynamics; peer and social relationships; and how they obtain information in the home.

Each interview was videotaped and later transcribed into English text for data analysis. Coincidentally, each deaf interviewee used either ASL or Sign exclusively. Six of the twelve hearing siblings knew sign. During the interview the hearing siblings mostly spoke English, though occasionally signs and gestures were added. In addition to transcribing, the authors of this book added journal comments to the transcripts. Our journals encompass personal and emotionally triggered comments to something the interviewee said that connected either to our own experiences as siblings or something we knew happened to family members or friends.

We've used the qualitative approach to analyze the interviews. Compiling statistical data were not our intention. The identification and categorization of major themes in the data were developed using a qualitative coding system. If we could identify specific behaviors or strategies siblings used to cement their bonds, then parents and others could follow their model, attending to how the opportunities for positive sibling relations were either nurtured or obstructed. For the first time, qualitative data collected led us to identify the critical roles in families with deaf and hearing siblings. Foremost, how well do deaf and hearing siblings really know one another?

We designed this book with a personal agenda: to get conversations going no matter where we are in our relationship with our sibling. We begin with what makes us siblings, setting the path leading to understanding the profound history of the 1880 Conference of Milan that changed the lives of many siblings' families for many decades. The stories of siblings represent the multifaceted dimensions of deaf-hearing sibling interactions—where conversations occur. Though siblings' identities are disguised through the use of pseudonyms, their families, educational policies and historical events have shaped these siblings' conversations.

All traditions have their way of telling stories. "Solo Dining While Growing Up," "Dam of Tears" and "The Siblings We Could Be" divide the text into sections which set the tone in providing an inside look at the emotional upheavals drawn from conversations at family gatherings between siblings. Throughout the text, as two siblings who live within, in between, or outside of the DEAF-WORLD, we will share our personal and professional experiences.

Aware that we might both be getting into dangerous personal territory, with unresolved sibling issues in our own lives, we walked into each interview believing the relationship between sisters and brothers is almost sacred, bringing each individual's cherished dreams, hopes, fears and above all, love. Our years of experience working with deaf children and adults, using relevant research, and employing analysis and in-depth knowledge of deaf history, will show how siblings' family experiences have been molded by centuries of society's oppression. We readily admit we are not immune to our partiality, which, like that of other insider researchers, is a crucial element in each interview. "Although there are many reasons to question the reliability and the validity of insider research, I make no apologies. It was our shared history that provided the key" (Preston 1994, 5). Since Marla has hearing siblings and Judy grew up with a deaf brother, we celebrated the premise that we too, are siblings. As sibling researchers, we were compelled to heed the pleas of Martha Sheridan, a deaf professor of Social Work at Gallaudet University, that researchers

> respect the participation of the people it seeks to understand ... if we truly want to comprehend the multiple meanings of being deaf or hard of hearing. This direction is critical if we want to gain insight into the meanings and experiences that children derive from the policies, programs, philosophies, attitudes, relationships, and other environmental elements that society presents to them [Sheridan 2001, 224].

As authors, we are extremely sensitive—working every step of the way to ensure that the siblings interviewed were given a fair chance for equal, well-balanced deaf and hearing perspectives. Perspectives from deaf individuals have rarely been heeded, a consequence of the stigma associated with being deaf, which leads to patronization, language and cultural differences, and the deaf community's isolation from the mainstream society. More profound are the cultural mannerisms, tendencies, and communication expectations each of us brings to the development of this book: The deaf researcher's world understanding is largely seen through her eyes. The hearing researcher has auditory experiences added to the visual. Our experiences appear to be defined by our hearing status, yet we have discovered that it can be irrelevant. The twenty-two siblings taught us that being a sibling, with all of its highs and lows, transcended and outweighed the divide.

Historically, we've read well-intended solo researchers whose efforts to study deaf and hearing siblings have given only one side of the picture, most often the hearing perspective. Slesser, who worked alone, studied deaf and hearing siblings using a mailed questionnaire with hearing siblings and British Sign Language (BSL) to convey the written questionnaire to the deaf siblings, transcribing the deaf siblings' signed responses (Slesser 1994). In contrast, our interview process entailed lengthy conversations with our interviewees. Despite Slesser's methods, our research supports her findings: the isolation deaf adults experience in their families, and their hearing siblings' regrets at not having sign skills to communicate effectively with their deaf siblings, resulted in ineffective rapport between the siblings (Slesser 1994). No existing studies have used both deaf and hearing sibling "insiders" to gain access to the thoughts and experiences of deaf and hearing siblings by using qualitative methods and phenomenological interviews.

The common threads we uncovered from the interviews will be found in the fictionalized stories, in the vein of new journalism, similar to that used by other scholars to show the complexities and deep emotions that bind siblings to one another or drive them apart (Feiges 2004, Verghese 2009). Each fictionalized story is prefaced or followed by text, highlighting the key elements, themes, and strategies of that particular sibling dynamic—in relation to the general set. Although there is a great deal of individuality in everyone's story, we all can identify ourselves in their lives in one way or another.

The sibling relationships vary in their intensity. Some of us may be buddies while others may feel we are missing something in our lives having to do with a sibling. Many have the desire to move to a closer sibling relationship. Our intention is to be the pebble, rippling into siblings' lives, to engage one another in conversations. The tools we discovered, from the interviews with deaf and hearing siblings, are the stepping stones to have not just conversations, but better insights into what it takes to have meaningful conversations with our siblings. In this way, at last, none of us are alone.

2

First Social Network

"It would be easier for him if we were deaf but it would be a lot easier for us if he were hearing."—Trish

A sibling exists only because there is a first-born. One cannot exist without the other. In Marla's family, Julie's birth meant change. Marla lost being the sole connection to their parents. She went from being an only child to a first-born sibling.

> I was almost two when Julie appeared in my life. Mesmerized by her presence, I was not quite sure who she was. Bewildered, I wondered: "Who am I in relation to this person—my sister?" Only we knew—instinctively—we had a shared belonging to the same parents.

Like most first-born, Marla probably resented Julie's very existence. At the same time, as sisters, they had the potential to be instant playmates. The underlying factor that distinguished them led us, as authors, to begin our study with this question: Did one's being deaf and the other hearing have any effect on their play? Perhaps. But as we began writing this book, we found a more pressing question, based on interviews we conducted with other deaf and hearing sibling pairs: How well do deaf and hearing siblings really know one another when they may be living in different worlds, and if experts believe "siblings play a critical role in our lives" and *supposedly* "know us like no one else" (Powell and Gallagher 1993, xiii)?

To address this profound and recurring concern in deaf-hearing family relationships, this book will reveal the attitudes, mannerisms and interactions in families that determine how deaf and hearing siblings "constitute a child's first social network" and explores the ways "their early influence affects them throughout their lives" (Powell and Gallagher 1993, xiii). The in-depth interviews we had with deaf and hearing siblings have taught us this: there is a scarcity of meaningful conversations.

21

What is the significance in studying siblings? Since siblings are our first social network, other scholars have argued the additional realities of contemporary family life, making it essential to study sibling relationships:

- Family size is decreasing—fewer children are born, resulting in more intense contact between siblings.
- Siblings provide a source of support to each other over the lifespan.
- Siblings rely on each other more because of frequent family moves and difficulties in developing friends.
- Siblings are confronted with family disintegration and remarriage rates remain high.
- Parental stress affects the availability of parents to their children [Seligman and Darling 1997, 119–120].

Sibling relationships are indeed complex, partially because of the emotional attachments we're likely to have with people who shared our parents and our childhoods. Our lives are shaped by the experiences and memories from the infinite childhood interactions with our siblings. Certain memories bring out the best or worst in us because specific events or personalities are attached to those memories. Being a sibling gives a sense of belonging; it is the innate feeling that cannot be described unless you are one. To some of us siblings, the shared history is sacrosanct and the future of our adult sibling relationships is fluid and unpredictable.

> Sibling relationships are lifelong, unlike parents which may last 40–60 years, a sibling relationship may last 60–80 years. The sibling relationship is perhaps the most long-lasting and most influential relationship of a person's life. The sibling relationship begins with the birth of a brother or sister and continues throughout a person's lifetime [Powell and Gallagher 1993, 16].

On the spur of moment, two adult siblings reminiscing about their childhoods, Gavin chuckled as he shared this memory:

> When I was about 15 years old, I wanted to call a girl for a date. So I sat down with my younger sister who was nine, and told her I'd pay her $1 if she'd call this girl for me, and ask her out. "Whooo! One dollar! Sure!" She eagerly jumped at it since a dollar was a lot of money to her. As soon as she dialed the number, it seemed the girl wasn't interested. My sister hung up. I didn't have the money to pay her but a few years ago my sister and I were talking about it and she said I owed her $5. I was taken aback and asked why $5, the deal was $1. She said she included the interest charges!

The above entails a common exchange: older sibling bribing younger sibling. We also pictured it a humorous tale about money owed. Do we go further, looking at the possibility of the older sibling's need for access as the catalyst for creating a deaf and hearing sibling interaction?

Entwined in many childhood memories are revelations of ways birth order influences the interactions siblings have with one another. A theory proposed by Adler states the birth order influence on a child's personality depends on the child's internal processing (nature) and external family social environment (nurture), not the sequence of their birth (Guilbeau 2012). In the case of Marla's family, her sister Julie reflected on how their family dealt with a deaf child:

> I think my sister being deaf has impacted our family greatly. The roles of older sibling were blurry because I felt great responsibility for her and my little brother even though she was the oldest. Yet I think I had a bigger case of middle child syndrome because of the excessive attention my sister needed from my parents.

Is Marla's being deaf the target or notably the culprit for Julie's blurred boundaries? Scholars have identified the tendencies with the middle child when they "do not have the spotlight" and "can be resigned in their position in the family even though they feel forgotten" (Guilbeau 2012). Regardless of the source, Julie's being younger than Marla supports the research conducted since Adler's time, where "birth order gets a lot more complicated in situations where there are adopted children, step-children, half-brothers or half-sisters, or where one of the children is physically, mentally or emotionally disabled" (It's My Life. Family, Birth Order: What Is "Birth Order"?, n.d.). While the blurred boundaries may be the reality, the dangers of role reversals could potentially set precedents that damage and disrupt sibling bonds, preventing them from healing. These sisters provide an example of but one of many families in which the perception of having a deaf family member overshadows underlying family issues. All siblings feel they deserve equal importance and value in their nuclear family to sustain relationships within the family constellation. Common family issues such as sibling rivalry, parental favoritism or caring for an elderly grandparent may end up as distractions, interfering with the siblings' progressive bond development. The deaf issue is no different because it is perceived as pervasive. The burden makes it nearly impossible for siblings who aspire to treat one another as equals to succeed.

As divorce and remarriage became the norm, some were the youngest of their parents' first marriage but older than their step-siblings. The traditional meaning of birth order rarely applies. If the shift in focus was the disability of the sibling, it may also support the rationale for making birth order irrelevant too. Tackling the disability label is the sibling's identity based on hearing status—deaf or hearing. The underlying message is more than what the label entails, as we will discuss throughout the book; but for now, both deaf and hearing siblings we interviewed have the disability label attached: the deaf sibling is living with the disability. The hearing sibling is the witness to the experience, directly and indirectly, depending on the circumstances.

Regardless of the hearing status, siblings have unspoken expectations for one another based on birth order. Few ever divulge wishes about what they think their sibling ought to be. During one of the interviews, Adele whined her deaf brother "*was never an older brother to me*" like her friends' older brothers. Ordinarily older siblings take care of younger ones, but in some families, hearing status of younger siblings trumped the responsibility that usually comes with being the older sibling. Although several siblings interviewed were the oldest, their younger hearing siblings' role in the family was to "*watch out for*" them. In many families, regardless of birth order, being deaf was equated with someone needing care. Both examples confirmed birth order expectations had no value when the disability label triumphed and the hearing status suddenly had the upper hand.

Nevertheless, even before a sibling arrives, the oldest child envisions what it may mean to have and to be a sibling. Parents tell their first child, "You're going to be a big brother (or sister)," "Mommy's going to have a sister for you," "You can help diaper the baby." Indeed, the reality is quite different, as oldest children realize sharing is required. They will share not only parents but often bedrooms, toys, clothes and numerous aspects of their lives.

How do siblings' relationships evolve? For centuries, scholars have studied family systems and siblings, in many disciplines: psychology, developmental studies, sociology and, most recently, disability studies. Beyond explaining the dynamics of sibling interactions, what is considered the essential feature of the sibling relationship?

> Simply put, siblings are socialization agents. From these social interactions, the child develops a foundation for later learning and personality development. Experiences in the areas of sex-role, moral and motor and language development are all found in the context of social interactions [Powell and Gallagher 1993, 14–15].

Let's go back to our earliest sibling memories. Social interactions have taken many different forms:

- She hit me.
- Why can't I go to the party and come home at 11:00? When he was my age, he could stay out. Why not me?
- Let's play house. You can be the mommy and I'll be the sister.
- Let's go over the menu for Thanksgiving and figure out who's bringing what.

- He's not playing fair. It's my turn.
- You better watch out! My big brother will beat you up if you even look at me!
- Please show me how to do this geometry homework. I'll let you wear my pink shirt tomorrow.
- Are you free this Sunday? I've got extra tickets for the football game.

The familiarity of these phrases stems from the roles siblings commonly take on within their immediate families. Attributes such as "Sam is the moody child," "Joan is good with money," or "Steven is the dancer" tend to develop over many years, change, get refined and sculpted by their experiences with one another and, as they mature, the outside world. In retrospect, the roles adopted during childhood may hinder or foster adult relationships.

Sounds Dominate

"Tell Me What You Hear," a game like charades, is a playful tactic used by a sister pair, Kay and Bree, to explore sounds, often a taboo topic between deaf and hearing people. More often than not, these discussions create a wall, dividing families rather than uniting them. In many instances, deaf people's learning of sounds has been confined to detested speech therapy lessons, family members' criticism of improper word pronunciation, or warnings about making noises. In the following fictionalized story, the abundance of sounds was inconceivable to Kay; she couldn't imagine they even existed. Bree showed her how the world is, indeed, steeped in sound.

The homecoming football game had just ended and they had more than an hour's drive ahead of them. Kay and Bree were getting restless in the back seat of the car.

"Hey Bree. Let's play 'Tell Me What You Hear.'"

"Ok, you know Ian's opening up a hard candy and I can hear the paper crinkling."

"Really? What does it sound like? High? Low?"

"It's a bunch of high pitched sounds all mixed together. You know how you can feel the paper in your hands as you crunch it? Well, each crunch makes its own high pitch sound and together they are quite loud. That's why they tell you in the theater to open your candy before the show starts. The candy wrapper's opening masks the actor's voices. The audience would be furious if they couldn't hear the juiciest part of the show because some jerk was opening a candy."

"Wow ... what else?" Kay responded with her left hand as she snagged another knot while brushing her long hair.

"Well, if you'd stop brushing your hair I might be able to hear some other things."

"Give me a break! You can't hear hair brushing!"

"Yes, I can. I heard it when you hit that knot you just brushed out. I'll close my eyes and prove it to you. You start and stop and I'll tell you when."

As Kay brushed, Bree nodded, "Now."

Kay held the brush still.

"You stopped."

"Geez. That's amazing. What does it sound like?"

"It's hard to describe. It feels like driving on a smooth road until you hit the bumps, you know? By the way, did you know when I was a kid I thought I was adopted because of my hair?

"You've got to be kidding!"

"Yeah, you know me ... the only one in the family with dark hair and the rest of you had light blonde hair."

"True, you're right."

"Also, Mom used to tease me and tell me I was the milkman's daughter. That's how I knew I was different."

Kay's emphatic ASL showed her skepticism. "You mean you didn't know you were different because you were hearing and the three of us were deaf? Isn't that obvious too?"

"Yeah, you're right, but to me, it didn't matter because all I wanted to do was be like you. You're the coolest sister. I love your hairstyle ... your clothes, everything about you."

"Yeah, you were such a copycat, but just kidding. Seriously, it means so much to have you in my life. I remember most when you used to come to my dance routines and we were a team. Remember you used to send me silly cues with your nods and applause? What fun we had together!"

Suddenly there was this growling noise. At first Bree wasn't sure what it was. Then she started laughing!

Kay's eyes widened with a quizzical look on her face.

Bree could barely get her hands to move. "Ian's stomach is growling!"

Kay's fingers flickered with disgust. "Gross!"

Like twins who have their own secret language, Kay and Bree were drawn into their bubble, a safe haven where no one knew what they were signing. As young adults, it was the only place they could be themselves, withstanding the potential for interference of sibling rivalry baggage: the undeniable differences of being older/younger, blonde/brunette, or deaf/hearing.

Since Bree has the privilege of hearing, she uses her advantage not only to describe the sounds but to encourage Kay to better interpret the world of sounds. While others would be reluctant to ask, Kay had no fear because she felt completely safe with Bree. Beyond that, Bree demonstrated that although sounds are unique and something to appreciate, they are not required to live one's life to the fullest. The obvious differences in chronological age and physical appearance were minor factors. In the bubble, these sisters chatted away without any reservations because it was who they were: budding adult sisters, sorting out their identities, unafraid to delve into what the other knew or experienced.

Looking into the early influence of siblings as a social network provides us dual insights from the perspective of deaf and hearing siblings as individuals who described their encounters with their sibling. None of us solely represents *the* "deaf" or "hearing" perspective, but this narrative highlights the perspective of individuals who live as deaf and hearing siblings, which has the potential to either enhance or inhibit their capacity to just be siblings.

We begin by exploring the patterns of family dynamics which is typically dominated either by sound or visual senses. Often family patterns are set by the parents and reinforced by the roles parents assign to children unintentionally or that children seem to naturally take on within the family structure. The patterns developed are based on how parents and siblings act in response to one another and lay the groundwork for the sibling's personality development. We see how they argue and make up; laugh and cry; tease and comfort; confide and keep secrets; support and take advantage; tattle and cover up; are generous and selfish; honest and dishonest; compassionate and insensitive; patient and impatient; respectful and dismissive; or can be indifferent and competitive. Consequently, adults bring unique, ingrained personality and character traits as well as attitudes and actions to their sibling relationship.

Adding a new sister or brother instantly changes a family's dynamics. In Marla's world, a new phenomenon came into play: her youngest sister Julie's hearing was confirmed. At nineteen months, Marla was mystified while witnessing Julie's responses to the sounds surrounding them, realizing what her sister was doing with her ears.

> Not long after Julie was born, I was given two big boxes, body aids, with wires going into ear molds that fit into each ear. Mom and dad told me they would be useful to navigate in the sound world, but there were accessories that came with them. I had to wear an extra piece of clothing, a strap that looked like a bra, surrounding my chest. These aids were bulky so my clothes were oversized. What's more, the sounds coming into my ears were unpleasant and felt absurd. The training was relentless; for self-preservation I developed my own rhythmic interpretations of what these sounds meant.

Julie, on the other hand, merely took sound in her stride. She loved the musical tunes in her ears. Julie played both the piano and the flute, but her practicing caused pain in Marla's body aid ears. Even when Marla made the transition to wearing behind-the-ear hearing aids, the ear molds squeaked and attracted attention, giving the sisters yet another thing to bicker about. To add fuel to the fire, Julie was annoyed by Marla's back-of-throat and nasal sounds as she was learning to talk. In spite of the sound battles, having no memory of first learning Marla was deaf, Julie "never thought of it as strange and it had always been a part of my life."

In contrast to Marla's being the oldest, Judy was the youngest of three siblings. Regardless of the six-year gap, she learned early on how to get her older brother Larry's attention:

> I had to flash the lights, stomp on the floor, bang on the table, wave my hands or touch his shoulders lightly. Waking him up was an occasional challenge; I would tap him, then move quickly to duck out of the way; he tended to flail his arms when he woke up.

Marla and Judy lived in families where sound was pervasive and dominant. Each family consisted of an older deaf sibling with two younger hearing siblings, yet the way the two families perceived their deaf member was vastly different, setting the tone and the precedent for how these siblings' relationships evolved. Marla considered using one's hearing as a privilege, not a birthright:

> Privilege is something one enjoys that is systematically denied to others. The ones receiving the privileges often don't realize it due to society's continuous cycle of how one receives special advantages. It's something that many take for granted until the privileges have been lost, taken away, or blatantly pointed out [Tuccoli 2008].

In her family, Marla was captivated by the power of sounds and the privileges it afforded her hearing family members. In this setting, Marla was also mystified by the ways people used hearing: to identify sounds, to communicate and convey ideas, to retrieve information or do so much more than meets the eye.

Hearing even determined how people engage in-group activities: to decide when somebody had a turn. To keep up with the fast-paced chattering lips, many deaf people were constantly challenged, relentlessly using their eyes to anticipate the movements. In order to overcome the overwhelming task of deciphering the mumbling, the strategy was to study the facial expressions, lip movements, and body language, and live by their intuitions. If circumstances led them to ask a trusted family member to repeat what someone said, the dependency for communication access became a constant reminder of who they were: a deafie. As a sibling, Marla's experiences revealed the beginning of a crux and the complexities of a deaf-hearing sibling relationship:

> Fortunately at an early age, I was so ecstatic that I found a place I belonged: the DEAF-WORLD. I had not only met and befriended these kids but I relished my connection to them. We were granted and shared the same fate in life to be who we are—as George Veditz used to say, "People of the Eye." Those brief three years with classmates at Lexington left a lasting impression on me. But, at the same time I was heart-broken—Julie, my flesh and blood, wasn't one of us.

Differences, Indifference or Acceptance?

It was at the Lexington School for the Deaf in New York City, where Judy interned as part of her graduate work to be a teacher of the deaf, that she experienced culture shock. The deaf students had nothing in common with her deaf brother, his deaf wife or their deaf friends. During that time, the Lexington students struggled to communicate and were barely literate. Although

Judy knew her brother was different from the rest of the family, at home the difference meant it was a way of life that just was. At Lexington, the chasm between the deaf children and the hearing world was a negative thing that had to be *overcome*; that dynamic never existed in her family at home.

How do these different views of difference come to be? Perhaps, if one does not fear difference anymore, it can be quite liberating.

It was a gorgeous spring day in 1974, blue skies, puffy clouds with all the trees in full bloom. My friend and I were headed for lunch in Ridgewood, New Jersey, an elegant town, its streets lined with designer boutiques and delicious eateries. Our four preschoolers were with us, the older ones walking alongside their younger sibling's strollers.

Suddenly, we heard and saw Tommy yelling and pointing, "Mommy, mommy, mommy, what're those sticks that man is walking with?" Our eyes followed his fingers pointing across the street, where we couldn't miss a man using forearm crutches, his arms leaning into cuffs while his fingers held the grips. He leaned each metal crutch one way and then the other, as he lurched forward.

Sue smacked her hand over Tommy's mouth as she whispered firmly, "Don't talk like that." I was appalled by her response. I spoke in a calm voice. "Tommy, that man needs help walking and those braces help him walk. Just like Mira and Lori are in strollers because the restaurant is too far for them to walk, that man uses crutches to help him walk to where he's going. Ok?"

"Oh, can we get ice cream now?" replied Tommy.

As a parent, Judy saw how other people responded negatively to people who were different, how a child's uncensored comments brought discomfort, embarrassment, and shame to her friend. Siblings naturally notice differences between themselves and their brothers and sisters: curly or straight hair, blue- or brown-eyed, athlete or bookworm, outgoing or shy. Are those differences perceived as the same kind of differences as walking with or without assistance, or as deaf or hearing?

Some families embraced or accommodated inherited differences as their norm, as opposed to other families in which the difference came with a stigma—a negative label attached—as something to overcome. The stigma, laden with emotional overtones, was a constant reminder that the deaf family member was unlike them. What each of us experiences as a kid, interacting with people of color as neighbors, classmates, or relatives, immersing ourselves in community activism, working in homeless shelters, or the kind that brings us out of our comfort zones, shapes how we tackle the differences. Unlike Sue, another parent described raising a deaf daughter in Andrew Solomon's *Far From the Tree,* said: "My whole life prepared me to access the Deaf world, and I am preparing her to be comfortable in all the non–Deaf worlds. We have wide citizenships in this family" (Solomon 2012, 89).

When we think about our place in the world, as vast as it may be, we are all interconnected, yet at the same time, we are a hybrid species. It is not the membership or attributes that divide us; it is the sting of stigma at every facet of family life, as Marla describes:

> It is the daily instances where communication barriers were constantly in my face. Not only were they happening to me, these same obstacles spilled into my professional work as well, in the public and private sectors where I was advocating for deaf people to gain access to work, where opportunities were either non-existent or limited. Employers were either skeptical or wouldn't risk hiring a person they perceived as "disabled" unless incentives like tax-write offs, no cost job coaches and other "reasonable accommodations" were part of a package deal. Hiring managers were unable to get beyond the disability attribution, regardless of the skills and assets the prospective employee would bring to their company. Furthermore, in my counseling work with deaf people living with HIV/AIDS, the access to quality health care was solely dependent upon on the deaf patients and the health providers' effective communication, often placing both at risk when inevitable misunderstandings occurred regarding medications, diagnosis and treatment options. And there's more to the story but that's for another time. But ... I am reminded of Rabbi Hillel, who used to say, "If I am not for myself, then who will be for me? And if I am only for myself, then what am I?"

Similar attitudes towards being deaf were evident in the ten families studied. Why do stigmas invade people's psyches? In his text, *A Case About Amy*, Smith addresses how stigma leads to prejudice towards people with disabilities:

> We are saddened by what we see as "their" misfortune, pity them at a safe distance, and keep them there without making ... any effort to understand how they perceive their situation. No one would admit to hating people with "disabilities," but the prejudice takes the form of exclusion and isolation. Many deaf and hearing siblings expressed outrage at the prejudice they specifically witnessed or experienced as isolation and exclusion, confirming that eventually, pity saddens, mystifies, and eventually angers those for whom we hold it [Smith 1996].

Our attitudes toward differences are only a part of the spectrum defining us. Siblings (along with our parents) are our first "socialization agents." They taught us society's cultural behaviors and provided the social rules *supposedly* to keep us physically and emotionally secure. Although people with disabilities have always been a significant number in the population, they had been warehoused, out of society's sight. For years, researchers excluded handicapped family members in studies on families, focusing instead on how the child with a disability affected those who are labeled as normal children.

> By listening to siblings, we know that the experience of growing up with a brother or sister who has a disability is not easily defined. It is certainly not unidimensional. The experience is complex. Like all sisters and brothers, siblings

report that they have powerful feelings about their siblings. Whether positive or negative, we have yet to meet a sibling who reported that the experience did not in some way influence his or her life [Powell and Gallagher 1993, 11–12].

Heeding Powell's suggestion to listen to siblings applied only to the sibling without the disability label. Others echoed his pleas. By the 1990s, practitioners strongly recommended support groups or sib shops to provide a safe place for normal siblings to meet others who had disabled siblings, in a relaxed setting, to share concerns, express their feelings, learn important information about disabilities and to realize they are not alone (*It Isn't Fair! Siblings of Children with Disabilities* 1993, Seligman and Darling 1997, Powell and Gallagher 1993, Meyer and Vadasy 1996). None of the siblings we interviewed had ever received formal support or even participated in a discussion with other siblings although several deaf siblings shared they had informal conversations with deaf friends about how they interact with their hearing siblings.

Why was there no deaf presence in creating these formal discussion groups? Like their predecessors who did research on families with disabled children, the few researchers who studied families with deaf children followed the earlier model by singling out the person who was different and who was likely to be affecting the family systems. Researchers have not yet considered how the deaf person was responding to their so-called normal family. Unlike our study, the relationship dynamics of past research seem oddly unidirectional.

Recent work has made some progress recognizing that people with disabilities are people first, with all the human attributes of those without disabilities. People with physical disabilities, mental illness and autism have become outspoken proponents of their rights. The main obstacles people with disabilities confront come from society's and even their own families' general attitude and treatment of people with disabilities—the stigma. The behaviors and attitudes stemming from stigma also spilled into studies of people with disabilities. Consequently, like the general public and many families we met, researchers earmarked deaf people as disabled. However, in this book, many of the deaf and hearing siblings we interviewed would spontaneously nod in agreement that things are changing in our society toward people who are different, especially those who eschew the disability label and live by the belief deaf people are members of a not-so-separate world: a cultural-linguistic group co-existing alongside the majority, hearing world.

3

Inside the Family

"I miss what my siblings are saying so I just follow whatever they're doing, like playing kickball or softball. They'd make archery arrows, I'd make one too. If they're building a house, I'd build one too."
—Jasmine

One day at grandma's house, at the age of nineteen months, my cousin and I were playing near the kitchen. Startled by pots crashing on the floor, she cried and I didn't. At the urging of our uncle, I then began the trek to doctors, audiologists and speech therapists; my sister tagged along. When I was about five, my parents placed me at the Lexington School for the Deaf in NYC. Three years later, administrators assessed the speech and language development of me and five of my classmates, and determined we were ready for public school. As soon as I transferred, my social network was demolished because Lexington had been the only place where I befriended deaf kids from deaf families who were like me but also knew ASL.

The depiction above of Marla's early memories is not unusual. In contrast, Judy's brother Larry, born hearing, was imitating speech and responding to their parents' commands until he became sick with a "bad cold" at the age of 10 months which, in retrospect, was diagnosed as "creeping meningitis" at age four. For three years their parents interacted with him by simultaneously pointing and gesturing, never suspecting a hearing loss, since Larry seemed to be a natural lip-reader. Larry also had briefly attended the Lexington School and was declared an "oral success." With encouragement of the school administrators, both sets of hearing parents—Marla's and Larry's—thirty years apart adhered to the recommendation that their deaf children were capable and ready to study and interact with hearing teachers and peers. Instead of entering a public school like Marla, Larry's parents sent him to a private hearing school with smaller class sizes, anticipating it would provide easier access to lip-reading.

Being away from home and coming home changes family dynamics.

Whether it is positive or negative depends on the interactions among family members. With many families with deaf children who stayed at dorms in deaf residential schools, coming home meant they would be isolated. Communication barriers are common among the family members, especially between siblings, regardless of whether they use speech or sign. In Judy's family, the three siblings found a way to rectify the separation.

> I couldn't wait for my brother to come home from his high school on weekends. We would stay up late, laughing and eating. He moved on to college and soon after he graduated, our parents introduced him to several deaf people and he began bringing his deaf peers home.

For the first time, Judy met deaf people other than her brother at home. The comparison was incomprehensible. Judy often didn't understand their speech, nor did they seem to understand hers. Even though the communication was difficult with them, Judy had also seen that speech was a constant source of stress, especially between Larry and their father.

> I was an innocent observer. I would hear Larry ask dad to "Pass the salt" but dad would insist he pronounce the "s" in salt correctly before he would pass it. It felt like he had to say it a hundred times. I did not speak out, but my gut knew that something was not right. Instinctively, dad's harping on Larry's speech and telling him "Never mind" every time he asked what someone said, did not sit right with me.

As close siblings, Larry and Judy both knew communication was vital to their relationship in spite of his communication struggles in their home.

> I wish that my parents and sisters learned sign language from the day my parents learned that I was deaf and my sisters were born. But that was in the 1940s, the height of the oral approach. I remember hating family gatherings and couldn't wait until it was time to go home. As an adult, I accepted the fact that I really could not participate at such gatherings and started to isolate myself by going to the TV room, reading a book or magazine, or otherwise finding ways to keep myself occupied until it was time to go, much to the distress of some of the family, who tried to pull me into the group.

Mingling with many family members can be stressful when there are numerous conversations going on simultaneously. Siblings often turn to their peers for emotional support. Like Larry, alone in a hearing household, Marla has many recollections of family gatherings interacting with siblings and cousins.

> Instinctively, I would often turn my head towards Julie, with a puzzled expression expecting her to lipread me as I mouthed "What?" Most often, she would keep me in the loop but at the same time, but I could tell she was annoyed by the interruptions. Anytime she got ready to explain, she would either say, "Wait, I'll

tell you in a minute," or I would get a one- or two-sentence abbreviated version, with little or no nuances to provide understanding of the ideas in context, the players' motivations or their separate contributions to the conversation. Perhaps my insisting on knowing what Julie took for granted potentially added fuel to the fire of our natural sibling tensions.

The tensions Marla and Julie experienced were also played out in Judy's family where Mary Ann, the older sister, played a significant role. She was Larry's oral interpreter: his window and guide in family discussions, with neighborhood children, with cousins and her friends when, as teenagers, they double dated. However, Judy, six years younger than Larry, could not avoid the angst occurring during family meals.

> Frequently if our parents were talking about their day, Larry interrupted dad, shouting, "What?" And dad's bark back was, "Never mind. It's not important." Without fail, Mary Ann jumped in, repeated the words, and often became the brunt of dad's anger.

Evidently, using a hearing sibling to fill in the communication gaps can be a double-edge sword. The deaf sibling is continuously searching for ways to be part of the family interaction while the hearing sibling either willingly takes on or unwillingly is compelled to take on the responsibility to ensure their deaf sibling is part of the family.

Retrospectively, Larry reflected on how their parents' expectations of Mary Ann affected their relationship:

> Although I was the first born, my parents put responsibility on my sister, the number two birth child, to look after me as though she was the oldest child in the family.... Yet we were very close during our growing years. I believe that if my parents had not put that burden on her, we would have been just as close and she would have looked out for me on her own without the expectations put on her and I may have been more independent and empowered at the same time without the expectation.

In Marla and Larry's families, the oldest sibling was deaf. In both cases, their parents directed a younger sibling who was closer in age, to "care for" the older sibling in a variety of ways. How did it affect the sibling relationships? The outcome was different: in Marla's family it had negative consequences, whereas in Judy's it had a positive outcome. Other siblings interviewed, where younger siblings had caretaking roles, revealed similar contrasting experiences.

Another layer affecting the interactions are the external influences that force changes in family dynamics resulting in either greater pleasure or deeper wounds. How might they foster or hinder sibling relationships? Communication is key, providing access to one another within the family setting, a never-ending imbalance between deaf and hearing siblings. In Marla's family, the extended family of grandparents, aunts, uncles, and cousins who gathered nearly every weekend, had plenty of opportunities to compound the potential for misreading one another, adding to the rivalry developing between Marla and her siblings. Furthermore, in her teens, their father's death, followed by the deaths of other close relatives within a five-year span, caused relationships among family members to deteriorate, which often happens when death occurs. Adding to the complexity, Marla's mother remarried, adding a second set of three siblings.

> The DEAF-WORLD became my second family. Julie moved further away, creating her own network of friends and eventually her own family with two sons and a daughter. Joseph initially became closer to our first cousins and now has his own family with his three daughters. Although Joseph and Julie may be closer, I know the baggage from our childhood still haunts us.

Many siblings sweep their tensions under the rug, forming alliances with other family members. Siblings may find a common enemy or join forces to share their similar beliefs or perspectives about the pressing issues going on in the family. One unique difference with deaf and hearing siblings' psychodynamics is how the communication tensions arising in Marla and Judy's households, like all the families interviewed, revolved around the deaf sibling's access to family chatter. As trivial or profound it may be, effective communicating is at a greater risk compared to deaf-to-deaf or hearing-to-hearing sibling interactions. What could siblings do to minimize the risks of miscommunication? The only tools any of the siblings had as children were whatever speech and lipreading training skills they acquired at their early education sites. Prior to 1880, the language of instruction in schools for the deaf throughout the United States was ASL. However, a movement to teach deaf children using only speech and lipreading, called the oral method, pervaded America and Europe after the late 1800s.

During the mid-sixties, most schools for the deaf used oral methods of instruction, where sign was prohibited in the classrooms. Judy, a graduate of Columbia University teacher preparation program, did not anticipate the communication challenges she would face, even after having met deaf people through her brother. However, behind closed classroom doors, many teachers used ASL, Sign, gestures or any other visual communication with these deaf children. Judy, like many of her hearing colleagues, was not prepared at her first teaching job at the New York School for the Deaf (Fanwood). Scrambling to communicate with her students, she discovered bartering, where she taught academic subjects while her students fed her ASL vocabulary, the tool she needed to do her job. As a result of using oral instruction or bartering, nationwide rampant illiteracy of deaf students became the norm. Back in 1976, a report by New York University's Deafness Research and Training Center stated, "Deaf adults generally are characterized by depressed reading levels, with the average 18-year-old deaf student reading at the fifth grade level (Schein, et al. 1976, 17).

However, many current education reports have indicated the persistent illiteracy is also compounded by failure of effective communication in the home.

> ... two of the best predictors of deaf students' academic achievement are parents' acceptance of their child's hearing loss and their having high expectations for their children. These two attitudes may be more frequent in deaf parents than hearing parents, but they need not be. Involvement in their children's learning and effective parent-child communication are what is important [Marschark and Hauser, 2012, 84].

As a sibling, Judy was forced to choose between her love for teaching and finding a place that supported ASL.

> My professional work in deaf education haunted me. I had loved the deaf kids at Fanwood but I couldn't go back there. I just couldn't bear the hypocrisy of the system. Yet, my interest in sign continued: With a friend whose parents were deaf, I trekked into New York to take ASL classes. Each time I saw Larry and Carolyn at family gatherings, I was eager to use my new Sign skills with them.

For ten years, while attending public schools, Marla knew there was a language that belonged to the deaf.

> ASL changed my life. It wasn't considered or ever used in my household. I was fifteen years old when I befriended deaf teenagers at a Deaf Teen club; there I was able to retrieve my memory of Sign and use what I learned from my hearing itinerant teachers.

Although Judy's sister, Mary Ann, their parents and other relatives continued to communicate with Larry and his wife Carolyn through speech and lipreading, Judy had chosen a different path:

> When I began Signing with my brother and his deaf wife, no one in the family objected or even commented about it. Sign just became part of our lives and was the way we talked.

In contrast, Marla's family mocked her when she first started signing at home:

> We don't understand you. Please put your hands underneath your butt. This is ridiculous. Use your voice to speak to us.

High school and college are the places where young adults begin to cement their identities and where peer influence becomes paramount. It is also the beginning of a gradual search for clarity in the degree of closeness with their siblings. Even as a teenager, Marla was intrigued by her deaf friends' stories about their hearing siblings.

> Some of my deaf friends saw their hearing siblings as their best friends while others cringed. For years I was obsessed with trying to understand what made it possible for these deaf and hearing siblings to be close.

By the mid–1970s, ASL was gaining recognition as a language, with its own syntax and grammar. Judy's years of increased Sign may have strengthened her bonds to her deaf family members; however, her Signing remained at a plateau level of English word order with missed concepts that a syntax and grammar would provide. By studying with a deaf professional and a native speaker of ASL, Judy uncovered a tipping point:

> My first class with Eileen changed my life. She taught the class without voice, forcing me to focus on ASL and not hear any spoken English. I felt like she had taken over my body. She made me aware, for the first time, that deaf people had a culture, a literature, a different set of values and experiences from my world—the hearing world.

Eileen Forestal, who coordinated the Interpreter Training Program at Union County College, used many tools: she showed videotapes of deaf adults using ASL. Through ASL stories and ASL poetry, deaf adults described how demeaned and frustrated they were at oral schools, detailing their loneliness in their hearing families where family members did not sign. Hilarious stories of their dormitory lives, where the deaf students were free to use ASL, showed yet another side—comedians, serious performers and storytellers. Eileen was not only an inspiration to Judy; she was a pioneer introducing the field of ASL instruction and ASL interpreting as a career, especially to deaf professionals like Marla. Since 2009, as the fourth most popular language among the universities' enrollments according to the Modern Language Association (MLA), ASL earned the recognition not only as a language belonging to the deaf, but a language deserving of study in its own right, like Spanish, French or German (Modern Language Association Press Release 2010). Deaf people began to work in an emerging profession as ASL interpreters, specifically as Deaf Interpreters, earning a national certification awarded by the Registry of Interpreters for the Deaf (RID). Their interpreting work presented ASL's authenticity: "In addition to proficient communication skills and general interpreter training, the CDI has specialized training and/or experience in the use of gesture, mime, props, drawings and other tools to enhance communication" (Code of Professional Conduct n.d.).

Marla's experience as a Certified Deaf Interpreter (CDI) in various settings such as Individualized Education Plan (IEP) meetings in mainstreamed and residential deaf settings, medical and mental health settings, business meetings, local, state and international conferences and civil and criminal courts have endorsed how ASL as a language can be as productive as any other language in making a difference in people's lives in large or small ways. In the world of ASL users and non–ASL users, Marla's lifetime work mentoring her students, colleagues, and advising families has been steadfast with this thought:

> When talking about ourselves, the world and anything in between we choose to discuss, whether important or trivial, there is this secret weapon: The ability to transform ideas into practical realities—whether you're deaf or hearing—makes ASL compelling and irresistible, putting emotions and ideas out there, all at the same time.

Judy's exposure to the DEAF-WORLD led her to heightened awareness of the juxtaposition of her relationships with her siblings, Larry and Mary Ann, one being deaf and the other hearing.

> Though I had deaf family members and had worked with deaf children and adults for close to fifteen years, I hadn't even realized there were two worlds: Deaf and Hearing. Eileen told us: "Once you've learned ASL, you can never go back. You become a member of the deaf community." As I examined my identity as a sibling of a deaf adult, I began to wonder what impact my becoming part of the DEAF-WORLD might have had on my relationships with my deaf and hearing family members.

Your Sister Is Deaf

Relationships between deaf and hearing siblings force us to recognize there is an existence of a DEAF-WORLD separate from the hearing world, though they co-exist. The moment a newborn baby is deaf, or at whatever age the confirmation is made, unquestionably the family is forever changed. What does a parent think about the deaf child? More specifically, how does the parents' way of thinking about their deaf children affect how children think about themselves?

> Stating that parents need to accept the deaf or hard-of-hearing child is an overly simplistic mantra without clear-cut operational descriptions of how acceptance is manifested throughout various family life events. Each developmental window, starting with identification of the hearing difference and proceeding through linguistic and psychosocial development levels, lends itself to influences that will affect identity development; this depends greatly on how families experience the hearing difference (Pollard 2004). The child's individual characteristics (temperament, cognitive abilities, personality, communication responsiveness, etc.) will also influence how the hearing difference is treated within the family context and beyond (Harvey, 2003) [I. Leigh 2009, 68].

These vignettes warn us not to underestimate the power of parents' words and actions on their children's lives. What goes through the mind of the siblings we interviewed as these words echo?

GAVIN: My father was sitting there and a man walked by and spoke to me. My father looked to the man and said, "I am sorry, he has a hearing problem." So, I suspected my sisters had the same feeling. There is something wrong with me. Something was missing. I was a defective.

DARCY: You know, it just makes me think how ... lucky I am. How fortunate my brother and I have been in a family where my mom learned to sign and my aunt wanted to learn, and she did.

NEWMAN: They had a deaf child and they had to figure out a way to cope with that. Cued Speech is great ... it can teach him how to speak. He can do this. He can learn how to communicate better.

CHAD: They discouraged the use of sign; they encouraged lip reading and my mother became a very good lipreader and she preferred that I communicate with her by talking and she had no difficulty reading my lips. My brother is a good lipreader too. We never signed.

If the deaf child is cast in a role set by the parents, does this mean siblings are destined to continue to live by their parents' model throughout their lives? Or are deaf and hearing siblings free to be themselves beyond their parents' beliefs and attitudes? Since in most families, parents are the first role models, the adoption of attitudes, beliefs, and morals internalized by siblings toward the existence of the family members who are deaf come with mixed messages— they are one of us *but* they are also not one of us.

The *but* implies something's happening in the family that isn't normal. Dale Atkins, a psychologist who did early work on siblings of deaf children, had parents asking, "'When will things be back to normal?' Since this never happens, the task is to create an environment for family members to discover a new version of normal. Life is different now" (Atkins 1987). What defines normalcy? Change is evident, but what is described as *normal* to one family member may not be shared by others. Although siblings may live and grow up in a household with the same set of one or more parents, each sibling's experience is unique and varies depending on how their roles evolve within the family.

The brunt of describing a deaf sibling hit home when a psychologist interviewed a nine-year-old bluntly describing her perception of her undesirable sibling:

DR. CARDEN: I heard you have a "special" sister. Is that true?

JENNIFER: Yes, she's special but it's not a good special. It's a sad special. It's not nice to be deaf. Sometimes it feels like I'm having a bad dream and I'll wake up and my sister won't be deaf. We have to sign all the time and sometimes we forget. It's hard. We have to learn so much [Sibling Interviews 1982].

Indeed, several individuals have acquired perspectives of their identity in the context of being a sibling of a deaf or hearing person. The examples from the vignettes show some deaf siblings are still wrestling with their hearing siblings' perception of them not as a whole person. Others have siblings who say their deaf sibling is the one who has adapt: the world is a hearing place, and that they see no reason to take on the attributes of the DEAF-WORLD. And finally, even some hearing siblings with deaf parents accepted society's view that spoken language is the only acceptable modality for communication, and chose not to sign with their parents or deaf siblings in the home. Discovering identity is derived from siblings' interplay, yet what masks the siblings' ability to look at one another as equals is the stigma hovering in the background. How can siblings be honest with one another in their interactions when there are so many unresolved issues: what language to use, attitudes towards being deaf, unlevel playing fields in everyday settings, among other potential factors invading the psyche toward a child or a sibling who is not one of them?

Studying sibling relationships gives us a framework for how healthy families interact with one another. In families, healthy family functioning stems from the harmony of their shared family experience. If both siblings are on the same page, through conversations, they have a better chance of moving to a healthier place in their relationship: "Clear communication is by far the most important attribute of the optimally functioning family" (Luterman and Ross 1991, 55). So what does clear communication look like in order to create harmony? As expected, parents model the way healthy families resolve conflicts and foster change and growth. Another key component of clear communication is the language necessary to identify emotions interfering with family harmony. For example, a mother would say, "Amy, you are crying because you feel hurt that your friend did not play with you." Or a brother would say to his sister, "I am furious at you because you did not give me back my favorite Gameboy." Since parents and children bring their own unique qualities and characteristics to the family system, each also brings diverse interests. Negotiation skills are also utilized to ensure resolution of the natural conflict arising within families because "It is not the presence of conflict in a family that determines its health but rather how conflicts are resolved" (Luterman 59).

4

Intensities of Sibling Closeness

"I have a feeling when our parents die, my contact with my sisters will be done and I will be on my own. I feel obligated to stay in touch with my sisters for them."

—Derrick

Judy and her sister Mary Ann had an intense interaction when they both were in their late twenties. Living in different parts of the country, they were rarely in contact, except for family gatherings.

Even when we were kids, we did not get along; we had totally different interests and it seemed different values. Later, at family gatherings, we "walked on eggs." One day, Mary Ann sat me down and said, "You know, the negativity between us is baggage from our childhoods. The things we didn't like about one another, as children, have nothing to do with who we are as married adults. I like the way you handle your children and I know you're comfortable with the way I handle mine. We enjoy doing things together like cooking, baking and doing craft projects. Let's dump that baggage and move on."

I knew she was right. We both cried and hugged one another. I felt like several tons had been lifted from my shoulders. From that day forward we became friends. We were a silly, giddy, fun-loving pair, who still recognized one another's faults but were both willing to put them aside for the positive things we saw and could enjoy in one another. If my sister hadn't taken that step towards change, by confronting it and acknowledging it, we would have missed the long lasting, loving and healthy relationship we had for over thirty years until her death in 2008.

Some sibling relationships tend to evolve over time while others stay fairly stable. Like all human interactions, siblings begin by developing their own set of beliefs, values and attitudes about how they see themselves—their gender, body image, personal attributes, talents, social role, or even birth order—in relation to their family members and the larger world, all of which influence their behavior towards their sibling. Expectations of one another during their growing-up years are part of an evolutionary process, ultimately shaping various degrees of intensity in their adult relationships. As with the two sisters above, at times the relationships may not be satisfying, but at other times they may be positive, healthy sources of enormous satisfaction. One way of visualizing the full range of sibling relationships is to look at the model continuum of intensity of sibling closeness, created by Victor Cicirelli and Deborah Gold (Cicirelli 1995, Gold 1989: see Appendix A). It is often used as a tool where siblings can identify where they had been in the past, are at the present, or aspire to be in the future.

As a consequence of Mary Ann's courage defining what she wanted the relationship to be, Judy and Mary Ann instantly moved from "Apathetic" to "Congenial." Communication and willingness to listen were obviously the critical factors facilitating the move to a healthier place on the sibling relationship continuum. However, what was evident is that these sisters had the foundation of their native language, spoken English, as the basic tool they used to initiate the communication and negotiation.

In contrast to Judy and Mary Ann's relationship, Marla and her sister Julie grew up using English, a spoken auditory language rarely accessible to Marla. Therefore, these deaf and hearing sisters were not raised with a "common language" as equals with one another, a privilege the hearing sisters Mary Ann and Judy shared. Nowadays, Marla and Julie are rarely in contact, feel somewhat indifferent, or even some hostility towards one another. However, they do attend and invite one another to their life-cycle events. Like many siblings over the years, Marla and Julie's relationship is functional, falling under "Apathetic" on Cicirelli's and Gold's continuum, unveiling deeply buried emotions beneath the surface of their interactions:

> It feels like a pane of Plexiglas between us, constantly preventing us from searching for opportunities to maintain a relationship. While we can choose our friends, we don't choose our birth family. Julie and I, like all siblings, have our share of baggage from when we were kids. I don't even know if we can generate a decent conversation. But, of all the people in the world, my sister is my first family. Why should I ignore someone who could be a positive part of my life and who shares my family history like no one else? A piece of me feels like I'm entitled to all of the things that define a relationship with siblings—not only with Julie but with my brother Joseph as well.

Battle of Sounds and the Visual

Siblings' presumptions about one another get established early, involving even mundane aspects of play. Interplay between deaf and hearing siblings presents unique elements. Deaf siblings rely on visual cues for affirmation of acknowledgment, a dominant force in accumulating intimate connections.

On the other hand, hearing siblings, accustomed to a world filled with auditory cues, *may* unintentionally create barriers that cause friction between themselves and their deaf sibling.

> Often as children playing outside in our backyard, Julie would run towards me, tapping my shoulder, saying: "Mom wants us to go inside." At other times I would call, "Juu-lie, mom wants you!" in as loud a voice as I could muster, and wait for a cue in response, often leaving me with uncertainty, hesitant, or bewildered. These subtle differences permeate how we'd respond to one another, potentially tarnishing our ability to anticipate one others' needs. It didn't happen only once in a while. Like a splinter getting embedded deeper and deeper, it was a constant occurrence because sounds were in control.

In contrast, deaf children in deaf schools cultivate their own natural ways of engaging one another. They used their eyes to tune in—to get one another's attention: penguin-waves, stomping their foot, or flashing the lights. Feedback was immediate, eliminating the uncertainties siblings who are deaf and hearing may experience. On the other hand, deaf children have powerful weapons they frequently use to cut off interactions, not only with the parents but with their siblings as well. Joseph, Marla's brother recalled how his sister used it: "I felt as if you controlled conversations by not looking or turning off your hearing aids when you wanted to. That was frustrating for me." Although siblings may use visual and auditory cues to control interactions triggering distancing, the willingness to leave the door open rather than shut could allow the individuals to achieve intimacy.

Luterman's study of siblings presents two elements essential to having intimacy in a sibling relationship. Intimacy encompasses distinct behaviors, reinforcing direct communication with frequent high-powered equal contact with one another (Luterman and Ross 1991). As children, perhaps they create their own secret codes, put on dress-up clothes, rehearse and perform before parents and family friends, or pretend to be a fireman, doctor, or a teacher—sharing their dreams. In their teens, siblings tend to be wrapped up in themselves or deeply involved with peers. Siblings are an afterthought—except when no one is around—the natural default companions. Eventually, as young adults, siblings may use each other as sounding boards for their shortcomings, faults or even untapped potential, and while spending time together, uncover and pursue common interests. As siblings leave the nest, they part ways, beginning new chapters in their lives. Even if for a couple of years they drift apart, what they take is the knowledge that their sibling is out there as someone they can turn to, if needed.

What to Do If Your Sibling Is Changing

When siblings feel they are waiting for the next shoe to drop, the tension escalates. Those feelings involve a tendency to search for blame, deny the impact of their flaws, or downplay the significance of their discomfort. A common occurrence of this phenomenon was seen when deaf siblings, who used speech and lipreading with their families, came home from deaf schools with a different vision, and were hit with this retort: "I know you prefer to sign. That's your right but it doesn't mean I have to learn it too. We've always done just fine speaking to one another."

The change in attitude and behavior of the deaf sibling induced a tidal wave in some families. Some turned against each other, lashing out with labels of rebellious, deaf/ASL militant, or accusations of non-acceptance of being deaf. Several families tried to adjust but remained unavailable. Alyce, one of the hearing siblings, admitted feeling ashamed, while most families took the change as having nothing to do with them, while accepting their deaf family member had found another home where ASL was the norm.

The backlash is the result of what many family therapists describe as the "blind spot." When family members take a hands-off approach to learning to sign or hiring interpreters, ignoring their deaf family member's access needs, their behavior inhibits intimacy. What if we substitute the sibling with alcohol or heroin addictions for the deaf sibling who yearns for the family to sign? Everyone is affected, one way or another, until families pull themselves together as a unit to address the elephant in the room. Minuchin's approach to family as a system says that families operate as interactive units and what affects one family member affects all members (Seligman and Darling 1997). No one is immune to family dramas.

The full participation as a unit with equal positive interactions among family members is easier said than done, if access is denied to any family member, especially since optimal sibling relationships take time to develop and start early, at home. Many of us take our siblings' very existence for granted, not contemplating our expectations of them. For some people, despite having a shared history, siblings may be people to whom we have no obligation. We could walk away, guilt-free, believing our siblings aren't worth our time or energy. Others have a different worldview: shared family history warrants the effort that brings lifelong friendship and love. Some are still searching.

Tuning In or Out?

Siblings have much to share. Learning from their collective experiences, we can begin to help other brothers and sisters turn a potentially painful, burdensome experience into a rewarding one (Powell and Gallagher 1993). The sibling threesome we met, a deaf-blind brother and his two hearing siblings, may be intimidating to outsiders, especially when conversation requires Tactile Sign, including fingerspelling, with hands touching one another, sometimes on the face. One of the sisters, Val, spent a lifetime experience witnessing how family members and strangers were easily alienated by her deaf-blind brother's presence, including ASL interpreters who refused to allow him to touch their hands. Without Tactile Sign, how is it possible for him to have access to visual or spoken information in his surroundings? However, both siblings, aware of the recurring isolation and alienation, have turned to one another for moral support. These siblings, Val and Rory, entertained themselves being playful and shared delight at family gatherings:

> We would have this other secret. He would put his hand on mine and I would tell him who was talking, and who said what, and no one knew. I'd secretly sign in his hand and you could see his face reacting. Then, I would say to him, "Turn around and look." And he'd do that to me, signing back in my hand. So the two of us are telling secrets, though no one can understand what we're doing. We still do it.

The differences in being a deaf and hearing sibling are inescapable: access to conversations requires commitment by each family member. Of the ten families, half the siblings demonstrated their unwavering commitment whereas others did not, or did so unpredictably. While it may be difficult to determine which came first, the chicken or the egg, those siblings who described themselves as having a close relationship with one another took access seriously and personally fought for it. It was as if being together and sharing the experience had more meaning than dwelling on their differences as deaf and hearing people. Addressing the needs of a sibling was presented as an opportunity to care enough, appreciate, and share the love for being a sibling.

The experience of isolation and alienation during interactions with family members, without exception, was a common thread in our research. It is only right we begin with a spotlight on Danika, engaged in a conversation with us, offering a perspective so rarely heard.

The isolation dam burst—in torrents of tears.

We never imagined the family matriarch had a reason to sob. Though short, she stood tall, with her white, neatly bobbed hair, Danika ushered each member in her family gatherings with gentle touches, softest kisses and a tight hug.

But she shed an ocean of tears, crashing and thrashing like waves on the shore. Not one soul knew, not even her husband. The pain she endured had been trapped for decades. This 70 year-old grandmother answered adamantly:

> No. I do not want to. I'd rather leave things the way they are, because we have had so many years of getting along and our relationship is way too strong. We are real tight with one another.

All week, the sight of her siblings, her children, grandchildren and a gaggle of nieces and nephews on the beach, had been breathtaking. But, on the third day, the illusion faded. She snuck out and cried all alone in the bathroom, unleashing a lifetime of tears.

Why hide those tears, Danika?

> I didn't want them to see me. I didn't want to spoil their party. But their party was my party too. Although I had to wipe away the tears, the deep pain wouldn't go away.

What was this unbearable pain, Danika?

> There was so much chitchat going on, I was overwhelmed and exhausted trying to keep up. After a while I just left them alone.

The final straw resulting in the flood of tears was Danika's sudden realization: "I deserve better than being alone." By leaving them alone, she had become alone: although her family was with her, in the same physical space, no one included her in their small talk. Their behavior reinforced the message she had received since she was a child: "Never mind. It's not important." But she knew small talk is what builds relationships. Yet she was exhausted from constant reminders to keep her involved in their minute-by-minute conversations. For the first few days, she sacrificed equal-participation for their comfort of rapid chitchat. She never knew the specific family details: her niece got the lead in her school play or a nephew got an award for his essay about his grandma. When the reality of her exclusion hit, Danika never even considered burdening the family with her pain. She loved them too much to care about her needs. She regretted this decision. In spite of having consulted with her siblings to hire an ASL interpreter before the family reunion, including sharing the costs, she chose not to act on the idea.

Why not, Danika?

I was not used to having an interpreter.

A lifetime of habit; although she had used interpreters for formal family events, she could not envision having an interpreter being at the reunion for an entire week, or even for a few hours a day. She never anticipated the emotional impact of *not* having one, three days in a row. Although she knew her legal rights to access in other settings and was more empowered than ever, she hadn't anticipated the dam overflowing in response to the isolation she experienced. When it happened, intellectually she knew what she needed but emotionally she wasn't ready.

Why couldn't you confide in your sister, Danika?

I didn't want to be perceived as the one to complain. I didn't want to be negative or pessimistic.... I wanted to be respected.

She respected her hearing family and their needs not to be interrupted, but she also eventually realized her interruptions were not positioning her as an active participant in the family camaraderie. It further annihilated her into the helplessness of her isolation.

How did you manage the first few days, Danika?

I did puzzles most of the time. I sat on the beach while my family caught up on each others' lives. I would just sit there with them. My grandson whom I love would sit on my lap and I would stare at the water while he fell asleep in my arms. And ... my husband ... he watched TV the whole time in the hotel room.

Although rocking the boat may not be in Danika's nature, how did she bury the pain for so long? We may never know. Sometimes the desire to initiate changes in family habits is greater than the willingness to do it, but it can also be frightening for one person to tackle.

Those deaf siblings whose families followed the oral philosophy never understood why their families, especially their siblings, never learned to sign. The deaf siblings intently watched their hearing siblings interacting with their parents, grandparents or other relatives. At every meal or family gathering, deaf siblings lived with uncertainty: "Will anyone take action to include me?" As adults, most made it clear to their families that oral methods were not working and a visual language was a gold mine. Their words fell on deaf ears. The totality of the deaf siblings' isolation did not hit them for many years until the pivotal moment in their adult lives when they found themselves in a language-accessible environment—the DEAF-WORLD—where they could relax, listen and respond with ease, using ASL with their deaf friends. Their anxiety and struggle to understand and be understood vanished. With ASL they had daily chitchats. Their confidence grew as they became valued participants in routine conversations and discussions with their peers. It was quite different from their home environment, where they could have learned a myriad of social-relationship building skills. The majority of deaf siblings' fury escalated: "I'm doing more than anyone in this family by speaking and lipreading and yet often you still don't understand me. And you know, I don't get what you're saying either. So, why are we struggling in spoken language, speaking and lipreading, which are laborious for unpredictable and sometimes no gain? Why can't you meet me halfway and learn my language too?" It's like the elephant in the room, wondering whether the hearing siblings had even an iota of understanding about the difficulties of lipreading and the amount of anxiety that went into their deaf siblings' daily conversations.

Even with the best intentions and regardless of the reasons, the recurring detachment from a family member creates anguish for both deaf and hearing siblings. The elephant in the room reinforces why conversations never happen. It is too enormous to confront. And we need to recognize that before Mom and Dad even became parents, historical realities were setting precedents for the emotional weight emerging in today's relationships between deaf and hearing siblings.

5

Between Marginalization and Human Rights

"I used to say, "What were you thinking! You're so stupid!"
loud enough that it would make me feel better but I knew she
couldn't hear it."—Petra

In the ten families we interviewed, two recurrent themes appeared, particularly in families where being hearing was dominant: isolation and alienation. Yet simultaneously, we also found an inviolable belief, held by both deaf and hearing siblings, that sign was a legitimate tool to nurture sibling relationships. Concomitant with the beliefs was respect and admiration for ASL. Furthermore, knowing and using sign was perceived by all of the deaf and some hearing siblings as validation for recognizing and valuing one's deaf sibling as an equal, not as a second-class citizen. However, hearing people are not only the majority culture but represent the majority of professionals working with families of deaf children and bring their own beliefs and attitudes towards deaf people to their work. Like those in this century, the families we interviewed, regardless of their hearing status, were exposed and subjected to the same misconceptions in existence for thousands of years, going back to biblical times: the belief that spoken languages supersede visual languages. Ironically, today's society has enormous respect for visual expression in art, film, and other visual media, yet when it came to the deaf experience, visual communication—ASL—using the hands, facial expressions and body language—was neglected and devalued as an unacceptable language form. The pervasive denigration of visual languages like ASL infiltrated not only hearing family members but also the lives of deaf siblings who were raised with the myth that sign would interfere with mastering the English language: English would be stunted and never flourish.

The hearing siblings interviewed who did not sign adopted the beliefs of the larger society about visual languages. They frequently stated that other priorities in their busy lives took precedence over learning ASL; however, we propose the Milan Impact is the hidden culprit behind their resistance. Families do not live in a vacuum but are part of a larger world. Parents were the naive recipients of educational philosophies, practices in deaf education, and attitudes toward ASL derived from a revolution in the late nineteenth century that continued into the first half of the 21st century. Medical practitioners clearly stated their goals:

> The HRP (Hearing Restoration Project) is a consortium made up of some of the most talented, creative and inspired researchers in the area of cell regeneration in the ear.... These scientists are working collaboratively and interactively with the goal of developing a biologic cure for severe sensorineural hearing loss in the next decade [Deafness Research Foundation News: The Race to Cure Hearing Loss in a Decade 2012, 38].

The medical and deaf communities are at the opposite ends of an argument defining the value of how a person lives his life: whether someone without hearing needs to be cured or be accepted and respected as a complete human being. In the deaf community, deaf scholars have challenged professionals and families: "To have a Deaf identity is equivalent to achieving a status of human being in the fullest sense" (Gertz 2008, 231). Since the medical community seeks to eliminate the condition, they claim they are not seeking to eradicate deaf people who are alive today. More than thirty deaf genes have been identified and through genetic counseling parents are given choices: To eliminate deaf people's future existence, thereby creating a world without deaf people.

Springing from the eugenics movement, the goals to cure the deaf spread like wildfire into families' lives. Siblings can gain insight into how and why the attitudes acquired are so deeply rooted in their lives, supporting and reinforcing their parents' language choices.

> The influence of Alexander Graham Bell was substantial in these oral-focused efforts. The eradication of sign languages and the support for, and dominance of, oral/speech-based means of communication and education for deaf people was crucial to Bell's eugenicist argument. For it was believed that, when deaf people had sign languages to share with each other, they were all the more likely to associate exclusively with each other and find, alas, their way to marriage. Raised orally, it was thought, deaf children would be all the more likely to mix and mingle and marry in the hearing world, thereby eventually decreasing (if not eradicating) the number of deaf children [Brueggemann 2009, 114–115].

Alexander Graham Bell was the key decision maker at the 1880 Conference of Milan in his mission to introduce his beliefs using his affluence and political involvement. More importantly, his goals were twofold: to prevent more "defective" people from existing in society, and to increase his influence. Bell gave the conference attendees the ammunition they needed to convince their legislative bodies to pass laws that would transform the lives of deaf people by forbidding them from marrying one another, knowing that being deaf was a genetic trait carried throughout generations. Bell's power, through the Eugenics Society, was directed at a vulnerable group that couldn't speak for itself in a way that legislators would hear. His power extended to a network permeating society.

Michel Foucault proposes a theory that power is in relation to how order is created in society. He identifies mechanisms of power that marginalize and stigmatize people, specifically *biopower*, which is "literally having power over bodies; an explosion of numerous and diverse techniques for achieving the subjugations of bodies and the control of populations" (Wikipedia 2012). Bell's efforts, through legislation, became society's "norm." However, in general, deaf people insist on marrying other deaf people, and in the United States the laws pertaining to sterilization and marriage between deaf people are no longer in practice (T.K. Holcomb 2013). Currently, Sweden is the only country with a law that requires parents of deaf children to meet with deaf adults and learn about their lives, prior to a pediatric cochlear implant (Solomon 2012). The deaf community is slowly attempting to navigate and escape from this type of power exemplified by sterilization of deaf adults during the nineteenth century eugenics movement or during the twentieth century of genocide of "defectives" performed by the Nazis, gene therapy performed by physicians, or Auditory Brainstem Implants as today's latest technology.

As if these efforts to invade the body weren't sufficient, the cognitive mind where language exists was the lasting target, as it occurred in 1880, when an International Conference of Educators of the Deaf convened in Milan. In attendance were an overwhelming number of hearing educators of the deaf who resolved to eliminate sign in deaf schools throughout the world. The reverberations of the edict lasted until the mid–1970s. For nearly one hundred years, schools for the deaf in the United States adopted the mandate that sign in classrooms must be forbidden. The full power of the Milan resolution was unleashed with the expulsion of deaf adults as educators, thereby eliminating deaf role models.

In 1867 there were twenty-six American institutions for the education of Deaf children, and all taught in ASL as far as we know; by 1907 there were 139 and none did. The fraction of the teachers who were deaf themselves, and who for the most part would be expected to communicate with the pupils in ASL, fell equally precipitously, from forty-two to seventeen percent by the turn of the century, and most of the latter taught manual trades. (Nowadays an estimated seven percent of teachers of the Deaf are Deaf) [Lane and Hoffmeister and Bahan 1996, 62].

The die was cast despite enormous protest from deaf leaders who, in response to the Milan edict, founded the National Association of the Deaf (NAD) to empower deaf and hard-of-hearing American citizens with a mission to "promote, protect and preserve the civil, human and linguistic rights" (National Organization of the Deaf n.d.).

Like a river overflowing its banks, the policies set in motion by the 1880 Conference of Milan and implemented with the support of A.G. Bell and his followers left twentieth-century deaf and hearing siblings with unresolved communication difficulties in their homes more than one hundred years later, straddling deaf and hearing culture norms. What they didn't realize was what Dr. Barbara Kannapell, an internationally known scholar and lecturer on bilingualism of ASL and English and the culture of deaf Americans said, "To reject ASL is to reject the Deaf person" (Solomon 2012). Deaf and hearing siblings never fully digested underlying issues stemming from the conflicting messages that parents, the education system, and the larger society were imparting about being deaf, using ASL and immersion in the DEAF-WORLD:

> According to Sacks (1989), the roots of Deaf oppression were formed as early as the 16th century and took a firm hold over the next 200 years. Deaf people were considered incompetent, inferior and incapable of abstract thought. Those unable to acquire speech were labeled "dumb" or "mute" and often institutionalized. Without access to communication Deaf people were relegated to the ranks of the illiterate, uneducated and menial labor pool. They were "treated by the law and society as little better than imbeciles" (Sacks, 1989). He continues: to be deaf was to be deprived; and indeed they were—deprived of the ability to marry, own personal property, receive an appropriate education and find meaningful work. We have since seen the ludicrousness in this belief; however, this focus on deafness as nothing more than a medical condition perpetuated the majority culture's existing view that " ... to be Deaf is something less than desirable" (Harvey, 1996) [Seiberlich 2004].

One deaf sibling, Audrey, describes her mother's dismay at her daughter's lack of hearing, exposing the persistence of Milan's aftershocks:

> I think from the time she found out that I was deaf, it was a shock. I am sure like others ... any hearing mothers. It was a natural reaction. I understand. I mean any mother wants a perfect child. When we got married, she was happy. But then, when I had children, it was awful. She thought I couldn't take care of our children. It seemed to her it was impossible. Her belief that deaf people like us can't raise children. Deaf can't. Can't. Can't.

Your Brother Can Learn to Speak

Can. Can't. The irony reveals how parents apply these words to their deaf children. She *can* learn to talk and understand us but she *can't* cross the street by herself, live independently or be employed, all things expected of children. Like the families we interviewed, ninety percent of deaf children have hearing parents, who most likely have never met a deaf person. When parents begin to explore what it means to raise a deaf child, primary advice centers on how to communicate with their child who does not hear. The United States Government Accountability Office (GAO) May 2011 Report of "Deaf and Hard of Hearing Children: Federal Support for Developing Language and Literacy" stressed the importance of searching for unbiased information:

> ... a family's decision-making process should be guided by informed choices and desired outcomes. Because children can benefit from **early intervention** regardless of their communication mode, knowing the range of options can help a family make a decision that best suits its needs [May 2011 Report of Deaf and Hard of Hearing Children: Federal Support for Developing Language and Literacy 2011, 18].

However, parents often get a one-sided view when they turn to professionals for guidance. The siblings we interviewed covered a sixty-year age span from their mid-twenties to early eighties. Like the parents of deaf children born in the twenty-first century, all plowed through similar ordeals the moment they received the confirmation the child was deaf. They were beset by medical professionals, audiologists, speech therapists, and companies selling assistive hearing devices such as hearing aids, cochlear implants and the latest technology—an implantable prosthetic inner ear stimulator. More than a century following Milan, these services have been marketed successfully to fix the hearing loss, accompanied by a lifetime of costly rehabilitative services: speech and aural rehabilitation therapy, audio-visual therapy, and/or cochlear implant and inner ear trainings. Consequently, parents were and often still are drawn into a whirlpool of events led by hearing professionals who urge parents to use products and rehabilitative services with a sole purpose: to persuade parents that deaf children's residual hearing could be used sufficiently to learn to speak. The GAO Report identified the drawback of parents' exploring solutions to communication barriers:

> Experts told us that parents do not always have access to information on the full range of available communication options. Several said that the first service provider with whom parents consult after their child is identified as having hearing loss can have a significant influence on the choices parents make, especially if they do not receive balanced information on a range of options. For example, if

the family is first referred to an audiologist, experts were concerned that parents would choose a cochlear implant for their child rather than continue learning about other options such as sign language [May 2011 Report of Deaf and Hard of Hearing Children: Federal Support for Developing Language and Literacy 2011, 19].

Simultaneously, some deaf adults tirelessly and relentlessly advocated for deaf children to acquire ASL, the productive language created by deaf people which like all languages, enables people to express themselves in infinite ways, on any topic at any time (Valli and Lucas 1995). Despite protests, opinions from the deaf community were dismissed as irrelevant. Service providers' powerful influence was held in high esteem by lay hearing people who regarded their goal as a noble quest to "help the unfortunate." For over a hundred years, the deaf community was unable to rival the well-funded, better organized, and vocal hearing-led service providers. Deaf adults were inaccessible, invisible and deliberately avoided by those who administered the edicts of the 1880 Conference of Milan. Since the siblings we interviewed lived the aftermath of Milan, all have acquired a variety of communication and language systems, unlike the standardized English language taught in traditional classrooms throughout the country. However, the hearing policy makers and administrators responsible for deaf education neglected the most critical component in a person's life: the right to *accessible* language acquisition.

> Kloss reports that dominant language groups may attempt to do away with a minority language by replacing it with their own language or by dialectizing it.... The focus of replacement of course is the children; they will be taught in the dominant language, admonished when caught using their mother tongue, and even separated from their own group in boarding schools so as to be assimilated more easily into the majority group. Sad examples of this are the replacement of American Indian languages by English ... and of the sign language of the deaf by the surrounding spoken language in the United States and Europe [Grosjean 1982, 29].

Preserving the Mother Tongue

In *The Language Instinct: How the Mind Creates Language,* Steven Pinker states:

> Indeed, because the deaf are virtually the only neurologically normal people who make it to adulthood without having acquired a language, their difficulties offer particularly good evidence that successful language acquisition must take place during a critical window of opportunity in childhood [Pinker 1994, 37–38].

Why do professionals in deaf education continue to minimize the impact of these outcomes on behalf of deaf children? Gavin gave a succinct description of how professionals were unilateral in the decision for language usage and the aftermath of his feelings toward his siblings:

> I really suffered. It's obvious, my siblings had learned from my parents' example. They followed the Oral approach—no signing. The doctors and the speech teachers told them it was bad to sign. The school told them if they sign with me, my speech skills would decline.

ASL entered his psyche—a potential first language was taken from him. Defending their parents' decision, Adele's argument revealed the extent of the Milan Impact on their lives:

> I don't know how he feels but I think my brother feels like my parents did wrong by him, by not learning how to sign, by not having us sign and not having him sign as a kid. But the people that I know or that we know as a family and whose deaf children are the same ages as my brother are all in the same situation, so apparently at that time, that was the thing to do. They weren't renegades. They weren't doing anything that was different from what anybody else was doing. But he can't grasp and accept that. He just layers on the guilt about it and that's just wrong. They did what they thought was best and what people were telling them was best. You know they didn't do it to pull something away from him or to have us not be able to communicate with him. He has not accepted that ... and I think that, to this day, is where a lot of the issues stem from because he just blames them for his situation.

Why do parents go to such lengths for their child to have the attributes of a hearing person? Even in the early twenty-first century, the families are still at war, creating opposing camps: Oralists, manualists, Sim-Coms, and Aural-verbal users. The 2011 GAO Report reveals how little has changed since the 1880 Conference of Milan: parents are given false hopes with limited options based on misinformation from experts.

In *The Politics of Deafness,* Owen Wrigley explains how both deaf and hearing parents have internalized the claims by the Oralists and Auralists that every child has a right to speech, equating speech with the right to language, believing speech is the only *real* language. He states that the main argument is: it is a hearing world and the deaf child lives in it; therefore speaking skills should not be deprived or ignored. Furthermore, from their viewpoint, since acquiring sign is easier, those who learn to sign will lose their will to speak. The ultimate goal is integration, defined as deaf children passing as hearing or becoming a hearing-like person, achieved through persuading parents to execute tough love during their deaf children's early years. Implementation of tough love meant only oral communication coupled with discouraging and disparaging ASL (Wrigley 1996). No one would argue there are positive outcomes gained from the communication between deaf and hearing individuals when deaf individuals speak intelligibly or lipread skillfully. With training, some deaf people have the natural-born ability to acquire these skills, equivalent of skills in logical thinking, creativity or performing gymnastics. The impossibility arises when relying on predominantly auditory methods not accompanied by an accessible language. Even Robert Ruben, a medical doctor and former chairman of Department of Otolaryngology at Montefiore Medical Center, advised parents, "Language of any kind, no matter what kind, must somehow be got into the head of the child soon" (Solomon 2012, 92). Parroting sounds with minimal understanding of their meaning or how to use them to express oneself within a linguistic framework is the evidence of a lifetime of language deprivation for the majority of deaf individuals who were raised without an accessible visual language such as ASL.

One pair of deaf and hearing siblings were casualties of the political wars of the twenty-first century. The 2000 documentary film *Sound and Fury* and its sequel, *Sound and the Fury—6 Years Later,* are rare examples that portray deaf and hearing siblings who were polarized surrounding the decisions to perform cochlear implant surgery on the deaf brother's six-year-old daughter and his hearing brother's one-and-a-half-year-old son. Though we are unaware of the intensity of closeness between the brothers before their disagreements about implanting their children, their opposing views had the potential to change how they felt toward one another. They grappled with each other's beliefs about whether a cochlear implant would provide their deaf children access to the hearing world and with ways for a deaf child to have a cultural deaf identity. In addition, the brothers and their spouses engaged in heated discussions for and against the surgery with two pairs of grandparents, one set hearing and the other deaf.

The brothers knew sign and the existence of the DEAF-WORLD throughout their childhoods. The hearing brother and his wife grew up interacting with deaf people: his deaf sibling and her deaf parents, respectively. The battle manifested itself around what they internalized as the bitterness and loneliness their deaf family members experienced as a consequence of their attempts to navigate in the mainstream. Being hearing, these siblings witnessed ASL's denigration throughout their lives and lived in a world that reinforced the belief that spoken language trumps a visual language. The deaf grandparents vociferously opposed the surgery, fearful their grandchild would be deprived of having a relationship with them should ASL and deaf culture not be encouraged and not given the same respect as spoken language. The hearing grandparents, on the other hand, believed the surgery fostered opportunities in the hearing world.

Ironically, the hearing brother and his CODA (**child of d**eaf adults) wife were in the rare position to provide a bilingual home—using both ASL and English—to ensure their deaf son acquired both languages to his fullest potential with support from the cochlear implant, highly recommended by professionals in the field (Leigh and Christiansen 2002). Why not give credit where it is due, given the reality that the deaf brother and his deaf wife use ASL and English on a daily basis? Yet in everyone's minds, once again Milan took precedence, with only an *either-or* approach. Not once did having a bilingual home ever appear on the radar screen of either brother's family or both sets of grandparents, though each family had the resources to provide bilingual homes with family members who are language models fluent in ASL and English.

Going forward with the surgery came with risks; there are no guarantees the implant would convey complete access to the sounds necessary to acquire a spoken language. Deeply rooted negative feelings, attached to their set-in-stone perspectives, ripped the brothers and their wives apart. To some extent, the sequel leaves the impression that some of the divisions have begun to heal. However, these films graphically highlight how the brothers' language usage regarding ASL and spoken English has been influenced by the popular misconceptions and beliefs-stemming from the 1880 Milan Edict. The ripple effect 150 years later has exponentially pushed the pair of brothers and the sisters-in-laws to find ways to salvage their sibling bonds.

Policy Makers Prevail

In general, hearing people, including siblings of deaf people, traditionally have demeaned ASL and signs from other countries (French Sign Language, British Sign Language, etc.). Many deaf people, including some deaf siblings, also internalized these beliefs when it came to using it with their own family members. In 1977 a deaf scholar, Tom Humphries, coined the term "Audism," to describe the beliefs existing in the Oralist and Auralist camps: "The notion that one is superior based on one's ability to hear or behave in the manner of one who hears" (T. Humphries 1977, 12). The film *Audism Unveiled* began as a class project at Gallaudet University produced with students by professors Ben Bahan, H. Dirksen Bauman, and Facundo Montenegro compelling deaf people to recognize that they were dominated by injustice in every facet of their lives (*Audism Unveiled* 2008). As a consciousness-raising effort to empower deaf people, the film contained many interviews of deaf people from all walks of life. Although the interviews revealed a lifetime of trauma from being oppressed, their body language told a different story: their constant internal struggle between fight *or* flight. The constant breakdowns of communication with their family members was a recurring theme, bringing to light the fragmented nature of the interactions between them and their siblings, parents, and other relatives. Brief moments of connections occur, out of necessity, but rarely do these encounters provide the stability to nurture acceptance, trust and love. Having resisted decades of attempts to eradicate sign, deaf people were consistent in demanding acknowledgment of their right to learn ASL, use it, and live by it. Unfortunately, the cycle of oppression and audism endures: 69 percent of deaf children, in the early part of the twenty-first century, still live in families who do not use signs (*Audism Unveiled* 2008). The film ended with a powerful message from a three- or four-year-old deaf girl: "I'm human, don't you get it?" (*Audism Unveiled* 2008). The premises of audism not only include oppression by hearing people of deaf people; it goes further into the psyche of deaf people: those who take advantage of their hearing and speech abilities in the presence of other deaf people. Distancing themselves during conversations, deaf individuals neglect to sign and slip into speech, disregarding deaf people who depend on sign.

The 1880 Conference of Milan catapulted those beliefs into a worldwide formal education policy implemented by those with financial resources to run educational institutions and government agencies providing services to deaf people: predominantly hearing administrators. Schools for the deaf throughout the United States adhered to the principles of audism: hearing educators insisted deaf children be like their family members: speak, lipread and use their residual hearing. Sign was forbidden, although deaf children naturally gravitated to it, picking it up from classmates, most notably native speakers of ASL, who had deaf parents.

> ... if communication goes awry, it will affect intellectual growth, social intercourse, language development, and emotional attitudes, all at once, simultaneously and inseparably. And this, of course, is what may happen, what does happen, all too frequently, when a child is born deaf.... The deaf children of deaf parents have a fair chance of being spared these interactional difficulties, for their parents know all too well from their own experience that all communication, all play, all games must be visual, and in particular, "baby talk" must move into a visuo-gestural mode [Sacks 1989, 63].

Violence is a common tool of oppressors; it appears when teachers enforce bans on sign, a common practice in oral schools throughout the twentieth century. One of the older deaf siblings, Audrey recalled: *"The teachers hit our hands"* with rulers in the classroom, adding that she and her friends used ASL freely in the halls, bathrooms, and most especially, residential school dormitories, where deaf house-parents were their ASL role models. When the rulers were no longer acceptable, other more subtle behaviors to demean ASL and neglect deaf students took their place: hearing educators fluent in sign who instead chose to speak with one another, in front of deaf students and deaf colleagues, thus shutting them out. More overt forms of oppression, physical and sexual abuse occurring in deaf schools throughout the country by dormitory staff and administrators, have recently received widespread media attention.[1]

In circumstances where communication barriers are the norm, deaf people are instantly positioned as vulnerable with potential for profound repercussions when it occurs in families. *Far from the Tree* tells about a father using his deaf daughter, Bridget, as his sexual prey: "He began to touch her, then forced her into submissive sexual acts." "I was the easier mark," Bridget said. Bridget's late-night talks about her abuse with her closest sister, Matilda, caused more heartache than the abuse itself, when her sister was unable to let go of knowing. "I feel that I let her down. That my problems and my deafness and my sexual abuse were a burden on her," she said, after finding out Matilda committed suicide. "I'd said so many times, 'Matilda, any problem you have, talk to me. I know I've got enough problems of my own, but I'm always there for you.'" Though Bridget has two other younger sisters, she hesitated to tell them to be wary of their father, out of fear of losing them too (Solomon 2012, 91).

Though none of the siblings interviewed related any stories of sexual or physical abuse, the interactions between family members that are dysfunctional are ripe for internal violence, especially when communication is one-sided. Speech and lipreading for many deaf people is a limited form of expression to defend themselves. Our interviews echoed what was featured in a French film, *In the Land of the Deaf* (Philibert 1994) where speech and lipreading were the only means of communication allowed during instructional time, which required wearing large box body aids, regardless of whether the equipment provided intelligible speech sounds. If deaf students stayed on campuses, periodical interactions with their families, especially their siblings, were limited to weekends, holidays, and summers. Educators stood firm, demanding families adhere to the school's communication policy at home. In *Women and Deafness: Double Visions,* Emily Abel exposed how mothers, the primary child-rearing decision makers, were especially targeted and pressured to comply with the experts' oralist dictates, through articles expounded in *The Volta Review,* the journal of the A.G. Bell Association, the oralist national organization (Abel 2006).

An earlier documentary film, *Beyond Silence* (1959) by Edmund Levy, a producer and director of more than 120 documentaries, was made for the United States Information Service and nominated for an Academy Award. The film includes a Gallaudet University (formerly Gallaudet College) student,

Judy's sister-in-law Carolyn Brick, portraying her struggles to pronounce the "s" sound in the sentence, "persistence spells success" (*Beyond Silence, Part I* 1959). In 2013, after one of her adult children discovered this long-forgotten film, Carolyn shared her thoughts about it with her family and friends. Her words echo the manipulation so many encounter with the media's stereotypical portrayal of deaf people:

> It's been a long time since I last saw *Beyond Silence* and I had forgotten how embarrassed I was by it. It took many retakes of each scene before the director was satisfied, as I was always trying to do it with an upbeat tone, not with the long suffering demeanor they kept forcing on me. It is disgusting how condescending the movie is ... Kelby, Gary, and Gwynne, please explain to your children how warped this viewpoint is—and that it was a common attitude back in my day, and to some extent even now. And make sure they don't think this is really the way I was then—it was just the director's perspective that forced me to act that way [Carolyn Brick, email, October 28, 2013].

Even in the early 21st century, not much has changed other than the terminology in defining the accessible language for a deaf child. At their symposiums, the A.G. Bell Association advocates for parents of deaf children to use only Listening and Spoken Language (LSL), an acronym defining their mission limited to using residual hearing and speech abilities. In recent years, organized community events hosted by numerous deaf organizations, particularly the Deaf Bilingual Coalition (DBC), Audism Free America (AFA), and the Deafhood Foundation have been a visible presence in the mainstream, targeting A.G. Bell's approach as audist. These groups encourage others to continue fighting against a grave injustice that deprives American deaf children of ASL as *the* visual language they deserve. In her blog, Patti Durr, professor of Cultural and Creative Studies at Rochester Institute of Technology (RIT), uncovered a "Bermuda Triangle of Oralism" situated in the Los Angeles area, whose goals are to perpetuate A.G. Bell Association's mission: Advanced Bionics (a cochlear implant manufacturer), the John Tracy Clinic (an Oral/Aural Only training facility), and the House Research Institute (formerly known as House Ear Institute, named after a well-known doctor and lobbyist) (Durr 2013).

Since spoken English was paramount in the hearing world, parents of the deaf siblings we interviewed also have internalized these audist beliefs. Compelling deaf children to hear and speak equated to normalizing them. In addition to the audism effects on deaf siblings, hearing siblings also tended to acquire their parents' attitudes and beliefs. One hearing sibling, Petra, reminisced: *"I begged and pleaded for a sister, thinking I'd have everything I wanted. And then when I found out Edie was deaf, I told mom to send her back because she was broken."*

To some degree these perceptions toward deaf people have been counterbalanced by a few recent documentaries: *Hear and Now* (Brodsky 2007), *Through Deaf Eyes* (Garey 2007), and *Deaf Jam* (directed by Garey, Diane and Hott, Lawrence 2007). Each presents a positive view of deaf people, supporting the richness of ASL along with how meaningful it is to the DEAF-WORLD. Each film was created by hearing individuals who have stood alongside deaf people as their allies. Filmmakers interviewed deaf people and hired deaf and hearing consultants, holding highest regard for deaf people's experiences. However, we cannot ignore the fact that these film producers were hearing and still had the final say on how to portray deaf people. When will deaf individuals producing documentaries have a chance to showcase their work in mainstream film festivals where their families would come to realize their maximum potential?

Like the allies in the film industry, parents are the natural decision makers for their children. As children mature, parents trust them to take on more responsibility until they show the confidence to be on their own, as adults. Deaf children rarely see deaf adults in authoritative positions that result in making social change. Films like the ones stated are a beginning. Yet, for some deaf siblings we interviewed, several of their hearing siblings continued to be skeptical of their deaf siblings' competencies and efforts towards independence. However, as Petra got older, her view changed when she described her sister's participation in a school play, adding, *"I remember being so young and so proud of her. Because it was almost, like, I didn't realize that she was capable of it."* Somehow, as a young child, this sibling got the message that her sister couldn't possibly be her equal because she was deaf. Perhaps when deaf people do take on authoritative positions, as film directors and producers, their siblings and others will go beyond the audist beliefs planted so long ago.

Historically, films have been used as an effective tactic to change people's perceptions and attitudes. In the 21st century, how can deaf people and their allies compete with the policy-makers? Currently, a nonprofit organization is one of many examples that offer hope through its mission by advocating that deaf and hearing allies take a stand at tackling unacceptable behaviors toward deaf people:

> Facundo Element is an organization that actively works to remove oppression and misrepresentation of D-E-A-F people through the means of mass media and non-violent activism. We stand by the transformative power of sign language [Facundo Element, "Board, Mission Statement"].

6

Molding Deaf Siblings

"On my first day at a hearing school, having transferred from a deaf school, my mother asked if I was excited to meet my new tee-ser (teacher). I asked, "But what about Julie, won't she want a new sister too?"

—Marla

In the early 1960s, hope and optimism towards being deaf were widespread in the DEAF-WORLD. However, resistance was led by predominantly hearing administrators, who set Department of Education and governmental policies, promulgated communication philosophies, and were the key leaders of deaf education in every state. Simultaneously, based on work of William Stokoe, among several pioneers in the field of ASL, linguists affirmed ASL was an organic language with its own defined grammar and syntax. The response by hearing policy makers was minimal and did not take hold for most deaf children. Many family attitudes, behaviors, or levels of respect for ASL remained immutable and oral communication dominated, despite the pleas of deaf family members and the larger deaf adult community. These policies and eventually a host of federal laws were limited to providing access to educational programs as opposed to the foundation of family relationships which are based on human interactions.

The 1970s brought profound changes in response to the segregation of families and disabled children. In 1972, Congress passed Public Law 94–142, requiring public schools to provide education for all handicapped (as they were labeled back then) children. Further expansion of the Public Law 94–142 legislative renewal was the "Individuals with Disabilities Education Act" (IDEA) in 1990, which drew up specific provisions for local school districts to place each child in the "least restrictive environment" (LRE). School districts became responsible for accepting children with disabilities and for providing support services. This provision had great appeal to parents who wanted their children at or near home. Opponents of LRE challenged the law, arguing deaf

63

residential schools were the places where an ASL environment existed, fostering language acquisition. They noted academic and social skills were nurtured through *direct* communication with peers and personnel staff, where deaf adult role models were rarely seen. They insisted that the deaf residential schools have historically been and should be kept as the LRE (Lane and Hoffmeister and Bahan 1996). In 2001, a federal law, No Child Left Behind, (NCLB) was added with the goal to close "the achievement gap with accountability, flexibility, and choice, so that no child is left behind" (No Child Left Behind Act of 2001). Nevertheless, as a result of these laws, deaf children made an exodus to mainstream programs in the public schools. Additional services were provided: itinerant teachers, classroom note takers, Sign or oral interpreters, and teachers' aides. Mainstreaming had its appeal because the educators and families were astonished and appalled to learn deaf children's literacy levels in the deaf residential schools were lower than those of their hearing peers.

During Individual Education Plan (IEP) meetings, school psychologists, therapists and educators would report the results of their assessments to determine the appropriate academic placement for a deaf student. However, historically these instruments were not standardized or designed to assess deaf children, yet they determined how and where deaf children would be educated—with little regard for whether the child had fluency in a language—whether it was ASL, English or whatever might have been used in the home. Among many reasons for the failure, according to various researchers on literacy of deaf children, are the differing philosophies among the academicians about how deaf children should acquire the English language: use ASL, Sign with speech simultaneously, and/or use speech only. The requirement for state certification to become an educator of the deaf did not and still in many states does not include proficiency in ASL. In the twenty-first century, two researchers, Jenny Singleton and Dianne Morgan, defined the optimal educational environment promoting an accessible language acquisition for deaf children within a classroom:

> In this new conceptualization, an educator of the deaf creates an instructional context that aims to build visual attunement, emotional understanding and competence, proficiency in a natural signed language supported primarily through engagement in "everyday talk" and some explicit instruction, and competence in multiple modes of English that are accessible to a visually oriented learner. This immersion approach includes teacher modeling and structuring of the children's development of linguistic and sociocultural competence in their worlds (both hearing and Deaf) [Singleton and Morgan 2006, 367].

Several deaf siblings who switched to mainstream programs expressed their regrets at not staying at the deaf school, where being deaf was not anything different but a readily accepted happenstance. Ongoing interaction and communication were valued.

In the late 1980s, Oliver Sacks, a scholar on disability subjects, warned of the potential dangers when considering placement of deaf children:

> Mainstreaming—educating deaf children with the non-deaf—has the advantage of introducing the deaf to others, the world-at-large (at least, this is the supposition); but it may also introduce an isolation of its own and serve to cut the deaf off from their own language and culture [Sacks 1989, 136].

Most of the deaf siblings interviewed, like Gina A. Oliva in her book *Alone in the Mainstream*, detailed how being the only deaf student among many hearing students did not make up for the ease of communication and socialization in a deaf residential environment with deaf peers, teachers, staff, administrators, and other employees (Oliva 2004).

Justin, married with two deaf children, switched from a mainstream to a residential deaf school, and reminisced on the power of learning through social interaction:

> One thing that's often emphasized in a deaf school is learning by osmosis. Suppose the two of us are friends, I'm interested in football and you're interested in baseball. So you talk about baseball to me and I learn from you. I talk about football to you and my dad tells me about football and I teach you what my dad taught me. Now with hearing kids in hearing school, suppose there are two kids talking about basketball. Each often over-hears other classmates' conversations, learning more about basketball. A deaf kid typically wouldn't catch casual conversations among hearing classmates going on around them. The evolution of knowledge from one person to another person—I didn't get that when I was in the mainstream school. I learned very little from my peers.

By the end of the first decade of the twenty-first century, these laws have succeeded in integrating eighty-five percent of deaf children into mainstream public schools (Marschark and Hauser 2012). As a result, several residential schools for the deaf closed and others were in danger of closing amidst decisions made by state level politicians and hearing administrators and policy makers who have minimal contact with the deaf community. If the primary concern among the lawmakers was the financial burden to society, then why are there so many deaf adult recipients of federal and state financial services?

> ... according to the Census Bureau's 2010 American Community Survey, just over 48 percent of 18–64-year-olds who are deaf or hard of hearing were employed, Senator Harkin said, "None of us can be proud of the overall employment situation for people who are deaf and hard of hearing in this country" [Gallaudet University>Home>News>HELP Committee Public Hearing 2013].

These are the long-term consequences of not preparing deaf children for today's society. How do policy makers respond to anguished parents who admit their deaf child struggles to succeed in a predominantly hearing environment with public school teachers who have little or no training to address deaf students' needs?

Jaron couldn't let go of his anger towards his parents for not realizing the impact of mainstreaming on his socialization skills, which he discovered, after meeting deaf teenagers, were essential to his welfare. He reminisced how limited his interaction were with his siblings. During his interview, he outlined a list of things he wished he had to avert the isolation:

1. Have an expert, a teacher of the deaf or deaf adults, either orally or in sign, who would sit down with me like a Big Sister [or] Big Brother
2. Send me to deaf camps, after school programs, or deaf events
3. For emotional support, have deaf teachers or counselors who sign to explain to me about the communication issues, socialization, [and] frustrations and advise me where to find deaf friends, not just a few, but a larger crowd.

He ended his wish list wondering: "Why am I the one who was in need for support services when my sibling didn't go to ASL classes? I had no confidence in myself."

Records have indicated how parents of deaf children navigated within the educational system through a system using IEPs as required by the No Child Left Behind legislation. The 2011 GAO Report reports the dismal academic results:

> Although experts suggest that deaf and hard of hearing children who receive appropriate educational and other services can successfully transition to adulthood, research indicates that many do not receive the necessary support early on or during their school years to keep up with their hearing peers. For example, according to one study, the median reading comprehension score of deaf or hard of hearing students at age 18 was below the median of fourth grade hearing students [May 2011 Report of Deaf and Hard of Hearing Children: Federal Support for Developing Language and Literacy 2011, 1].

Deaf children who leave school with minimal academic and social skills cannot be expected to be financially independent lacking the fundamental reading, writing and communication skills necessary to compete in today's global job market.

Meanwhile, at home, their hearing siblings were not immune to what was happening around them. Gila described with sadness how her deaf sister struggled with academics: "She's got a great imagination with Art as her muse but her English is very poor. She's always not been a good 'book learner." Hearing siblings like her witness their parents' agony and hear about their different sibling from others while their deaf siblings are the innocent pawns in parents,' educators' and society's chess game, all expecting deaf children to take on the characteristics of hearing people. As a longtime staunch advocate of deaf people who are part of a culture and a linguistic minority, Harlan Lane challenged educators and families to define normalization in the family.

> The deaf child or adult is not an ordinary dependent, as any hearing person might be who goes to a doctor, an audiologist, as psychologist. He is a stigmatized dependent. When isolated from others of his kind, the deaf child with hearing parents and a hearing school is bound to feel deviant. Why can't he be like other people and conform to the demands made on him— most of all, the demand of facile communication in English [H. Lane 1999, 88]?

Signing-Speaking Simultaneously—ASL and English

Parallel to educational legislation and the emerging ripple effect of ASL as a legitimate language, the next generation of experts appeared on the educational scene. They recommended using sign to communicate with young deaf children. However, instead of using ASL, educators and parents adopted a new philosophy called Total Communication. It was originally an approach advocating that parents use whatever means necessary to achieve effective communication and acquire language. In practice, it became a way for hearing parents and hearing educators to avoid learning a new language, ASL. One of the most popular methods for Total Communication was Simultaneous Communication (SimCom); it used the vocabulary of ASL married to the syntax of English, while simultaneously speaking English. Many educators believed Sim-Com would allow deaf children to see English on the hands and thereby improve their literacy. However, what the users of SimCom failed to recognize is that SimCom is not a language; ASL is.

The parents of the older deaf siblings (those born before 1970) enrolled their deaf children in residential or day schools using oral communication methods. In contrast, the parents of the younger siblings had an alphabet soup of mainstreaming and residential schools using all forms of "English on the Hands" known as Manually Coded English (MCE). By the early 1970s, professionals in the field of deaf education who created MCE systems had a common goal: to make the English visible to deaf children. Educators recognized that the longstanding use of oral communication methods was not resulting in literacy for many deaf children. As they further analyzed the challenges of lipreading inherent in oralism, they acknowledged that spoken English was not visually accessible to deaf children while engaged in conversations with hearing teachers, peers and family members.

As a response, these educators took the matter into their own hands to create visual communication systems. MCE systems entail an array of hand signals by borrowing vocabulary and the signed alphabet from ASL. Educators identified Signs to match English root words. Then, they invented specific hand signals for the to-be verbs, verb inflections, noun suffixes and pronouns, all placed together in English word order. Interestingly, the MCE systems differed from one another based on their assessment of those that preceded them. For example, Signing Essential English (SEE 1) later became Signing Exact English (SEE 2), then eventually became Signed English (SE); all were widely adopted by deaf education programs. Within the core of the deaf community, none of the MCE systems evolved naturally. MCE systems instead became popular among hearing parents and professionals (teachers, speech therapists, audiologists and interpreters). During this time, the majority of deaf children began attending day programs, often in separate classes within a neighborhood school. The younger deaf siblings attended these programs, lived at home with their families, and used MCE systems with their hearing siblings as well as with their parents. One of the selling points of MCE systems was the belief that it was *easier* to use the word order of English, a language their hearing parents and hearing siblings already knew, as opposed to learning the grammar of a different language.

If educators shifted their focus to creating alternative ways to acquire English, did it justify superimposing the features of a visual-spatial language (ASL) onto a linear language (English)? Since "ASL is a simultaneous language in which individual signs are amalgamated into composite ones; one complex, fluid movement" (Solomon 2012, 82), ASL incorporates the essence of the meaning where the relationship of ideas is interdependent. In contrast, in English, the word order of *The train hit the car* versus *The car hit the train* determines which vehicle hit and which vehicle was hit. MCE systems retain the concept that "English is a sequential language, with words produced in defined order; the listener's short-term memory holds the words of a sentence, then takes meaning from their relationship" (Solomon 2012, 82). For example, MCE Signers would use the invented Sign for *the* followed by an ASL sign for *train*, a separate ASL sign for *hit* followed by another ASL sign for *car*. What's the advantage of using an MCE system when ASL already offers equivalent meaning? In the early '70s, recognition of ASL as a complete language was in its infancy, still defending its legitimacy. In those days, trainings, classes, workshops or even assessments for ASL were nonexistent.

Since linguists who have studied ASL over the last century have confirmed that ASL is not a linear language but instead is a visual-spatial language, ASL begins with the signing space as a key parameter coupled with specific handshapes for each signed word. For every word, the ASL user needs to ensure his palm orientation is correct (up, down, to one side or the other). The positioning of the ASL signs for accuracy, identifying the location (on the body, the face and/or in signing space) and the movement (fixed or moving in defined ways) are all essential to convey the meaning. Each parameter reveals by showing, rather than telling, how each ASL sign and concept is interdependent. Non-manual grammatical signals (NMGS), also known as facial expressions and mouth morphemes, are additional parameters since they define the language prosody (the stresses and intonations of each word/sign). In ASL, the same two sentences ("The *train* hit the car" and "The *car* hit the train") would be conveyed spatially in ASL by setting up and positioning the ASL sign for *train* in one space, setting and positioning the ASL sign for *car* in another, and then moving the appropriate vehicle to show which one hit the other. Simultaneously, NMGS and mouth morphemes show the intensity of the distance and the hit.

As educators went down the path of using MCE systems, they discovered they needed a variety of additional tools to master the intricacies of the English language. Teaching deaf students multiple meanings of English words when ASL had separate vocabulary for each meaning continued to be their challenge. For example, Gerry Gustason, one of the founders of SEE 1, created a two-out-of-three rule determining which ASL vocabulary to use for these English words. In her example for the English word *wind*, where several meanings were to be considered: air in motion, or the turning of a stem on a watch, or the turning of rope to gather in a circular fashion, she applied the two-out-of-three rule. To decide which sign to use, the educator would have to first determine: Is the word spelled the same? (yes) Does the word sound the same? (no) And does the word mean the same thing? (no) Therefore, based on the only one criterion that the spelling was the same, they would borrow the two different ASL vocabulary words for SEE since ASL already had the different meanings for them to use.

The two-out-of three-rule says that if two of the questions are answered in the affirmative, one sign is used, as in the following example:

> To *bear* a burden, *bear* a child or meet a *bear*, are all signed with the same basic sign for the word bear because spelling and sound are the same and only the meaning differs. Similarly only one sign for *run* is used whether the meaning is John *is running*, the water is *running*, or your nose is *running* or the man is *running* for office ... the main reason for this was to represent on the hands what was said in English, so the students learned how a concept was represented in English [Gustason 1990, 116].

Regardless of her decision of which sign to use, the idea behind this tenet of SEE was to identify only the "signs to represent one English word each ...

English should be signed as it is spoken" (Gustason 1990, 115). These kinds of decisions were ridiculed by and saddened fluent ASL users, especially when they saw children from MCE programs Signing the equivalent of: "She saw a bare (bear) and her stocking ripped (ran) as fast as her legs wood (would) carry her." Another feature of MCE systems was the addition of initialized Signs—the fingerspelled first letter of an English word added to the ASL vocabulary—to distinguish between English synonyms like *demonstrate* and *example*. To Sign the word *example*, instead of using the index finger handshape as used in ASL with the dominant hand, MCE substitutes the fingerspelled letter E. For *demonstrate*, the Signer substitutes the fingerspelled letter D. This feature of MCE systems has been adopted by the recent generations of mainstreamed children who have been exposed to them through interacting with their Sign language interpreters (many of whom learned MCE systems instead of ASL).

The MCE system's founders had positive intentions—to distinguish English words using numerous different hand signals in order to improve deaf children's English literacy—but in reality, the research data showed the results to be otherwise (Lane and Hoffmeister and Bahan 1996). The MCE systems were designed to be used while simultaneously speaking English. Genie Gertz, a deaf scholar, explains several reasons for the failure of Simultaneous Communication (SimCom):

> A limited number of people are particularly skilled at talking and signing at the same time, but many other people are really not able to do it. They try to talk and sign at the same time and nothing clear comes out. As a result of using Simcom, many signs are dropped out. The sign also deteriorates significantly in its quality and intelligibility. Often, many Deaf people can't understand what people are saying, and they have to work so much harder to try and receive the message. When people speak English, the ASL becomes unintelligible. SimCom is an incomprehensible mix of two different modalities.... The language issue with deaf children addresses the fact that the acquisition of a first language is very important. By trying to teach ASL and English, Simcom confuses deaf children further because, when some people sign and speak at the same time, they are ultimately doing neither correctly.... Simcom doesn't work because ASL and English are two completely different languages. The underlying mechanism of Simcom requires the "speaking" part that imposes on Deaf people to use English, often for the convenience of hearing people. In this sense, SimCom disempowers Deaf people from using ASL to the full extent and consequently weakens them in development of their Deaf identity [Gertz 2008, 226–227].

SimCom eventually became the communication system in the home among many families as a result of the efforts of MCE professionals.

With ASL emerging as the preferred language by the deaf siblings interviewed, deaf and hearing siblings were left with a myriad of communication modalities. Darcy, who learned to Sign as a child, described how she communicates with her deaf brother:

> When my mom learned how to Sign, she probably took Signed English classes, not ASL. Sadly, I still use Signed English with my brother. I try to incorporate ASL but I know I am very weak with ASL. Pretty much, with anyone else who's deaf, my brother uses ASL. When he's with me, it's just force of habit for him to code switch from ASL to Signed English.

As adults, deaf siblings would code-switch by going back and forth between using ASL in the DEAF-WORLD and MCE systems with their family members. In addition, they adapt with deaf people who tend to use MCE systems. The act of code-switching, as this sibling describes, is indicative of those deaf and hearing siblings who are trapped by their communication patterns stemming from their childhood. Code-switching not only creates frustrations during conversations, causing many misunderstandings, it prevents both deaf and hearing siblings from becoming fluent in ASL as adults—a commodity both clearly see as being critical to bonding more closely with one another.

Parallel to the creation of MCE systems, other educators entered the fray in order to make the sounds of English words visible to deaf children, recognizing visual access was the key to effective communication. To achieve that goal, R. Orin Corbett developed a system to differentiate the sounds of English. Known as Cued Speech, it was described as "a visual mode of communication that uses handshapes and placements in combination with the mouth movements of speech to make the phonemes of a spoken language look different from each other" (Cued Speech n.d.). The uniqueness of Cued Speech was speech's multiple sounds that look alike on the lips or spoken inside the mouth or behind the teeth, are differentiated by being nasal, using one's breath or voiced. For example, a limited number of hand signals created would provide the cues to show the difference between mama, papa, and baby which look the same on the lips with their multiple syllables. To address the challenge with decoding during reading, writing and speech articulation, another tool was developed by the International Communications Learning Institute (ICLI) known as Visual Phonics in 1982. Its mission was to use tactile, kinesthetic and visual techniques to teach deaf children to "see the sound and internalize English phonemes and understand how they map onto English letters and words" (See the Sound n.d.).

Educators, speech therapists, audiologists and parents have seen some success using these phonetically based systems to teach deaf children speech, lipreading and pronunciation. However, the trade-off of the time spent doing these activities is the missed opportunities for ongoing engagement in conversations and fewer opportunities to develop critical thinking skills through reading, writing and comprehension. Sharing feelings, thoughts, and observations through interactions with family members, peers, and service providers is the foundation for any child's language acquisition. In their earliest years, siblings are supposedly naturally engaged in this process, assisting and enabling their siblings to acquire a native language: every child's birthright.

Research has shown that simultaneously mixing the ASL vocabulary with spoken English—like MCE systems—breaks the grammatical rules of both languages and muddies the speaker's intention and meaning (Gertz 2008). Nevertheless, under the direction of predominantly hearing administrators and other educational staff members, every parent of the younger siblings used MCE or Cued Speech at home, rather than exclusively using speech. None of these siblings were raised using ASL, the only visual-gestural system affirmed by linguists to be a language. Children lived the consequences of the professional advice parents received about language choices, but also have been affected by their parents' core attitudes to using ASL as opposed to using MCE systems. In spite of the history of Milan and its consequences, we asked the siblings, "How did you communicate with your parents and siblings as children and as adults?" All but one of the twenty-two deaf and hearing siblings interviewed followed parental communication patterns—whatever communication method they used as children, whether it was using speech or sign, they continued to use in their adult conversations. One exception was Risa, who used oral communication methods with her deaf brother while growing up, but as an adult, switched to Sign.

Laurel, an ASL interpreter, juggled between using both ASL and SimCom at home:

> When the three of us are together, we typically use ASL. My mom uses English-like Signing and ASL. When it's just the two of us (me and my mom), we SimCom. My mom did that because she thought that I would learn both languages, English and ASL. But she didn't realize that when you SimCom, you're splitting the languages. When I ask mom to do voice-off because I really want work on my ASL, she'd be willing but we slip into our comfort zone, Sim-Com, after a few minutes. And with my sister, it changes the dynamics whenever we use ASL.

The fallback to SimCom caused distress for the hearing sibling. She was keenly aware that each time her sister and mom were exposed to partial information either from lipreading, MCE or a phonetic system, their chances to be proficient in ASL diminished. When she studied ASL in her ASL Interpreting program, she learned for the first time the only way her sister and mom could be fully immersed in discussing complex topics effortlessly, including nuances, was for the three of them to use ASL exclusively. In addition, when siblings and other family members are constantly making adjustments and accommodations about which communication systems to use with one another, it interferes and distracts them from whatever they aimed to discuss, whether it's to decide where to spend a vacation or what present to buy one another for their birthdays, seeing one another's humor, sarcasms, hints, etc.—the very building blocks of their evolving relationship.

Being Bilingual

Since deaf and hearing siblings grew up under the Milan Impact, they bore the consequences of the edict banning ASL. Yet, conversations among siblings about ASL are a rarity. Most of the deaf and hearing siblings admitted they have not had heart-to-heart talks about ways to resolve their differences, largely a result of the limitations and frustrations, inherent in their communication using speech and MCE systems. Our research showed an underlying attitude toward ASL that continues to obstruct opportunities for sibling bonding. Conference workshops and retreats for families with deaf members, hosted by local and national organizations, are emerging with sibling peer support groups as essential components.

Based on the interviews, we created a series of vignettes of the non-signing hearing siblings and their deaf siblings as if they were in the same room. Although the interviews were conducted separately, these siblings were specifically vocal about ASL and its significance in the DEAF-WORLD. Since the adult deaf siblings have made a conscious decision to communicate in ASL, the scenarios propelled us to reframe perspectives of both deaf and hearing siblings. These vignettes uncover the non-signing siblings' resistance to the change their deaf siblings had embraced.

Although they are related by blood, according to his sister Kacie, her brother's discovery of ASL and the DEAF-WORLD is perceived to be the root of their conflict:

> Our relationship is so negative part of me doesn't want to learn ASL just to spite him. He's been trying to ram it down our throats since he learned it himself, after he was out of the house. I have a busy life, working and trying to raise a family and quite honestly, I don't see him enough nor do I want to. One positive thing though he's brought sign to our lives and I find it extremely interesting that I would love to learn it.... I will not learn it for him.... Why should I? ... he doesn't deserve to have us take time out of our lives to learn a language that is his. He's never tried to do anything that's ours. You know, he was kind of forced to and resented it and then resented us. We can talk with one another, just like we did when we were kids. So why do I need to learn it? So, why doesn't he make peace with that?

With the communication challenges, siblings have it within their power to embrace, resist or resent changes. What if Kacie's learning ASL isn't such a big deal? She is stating just because he's changed doesn't mean she had to when they understood one another perfectly. In our interview, her deaf brother Maxel had an answer:

> I feel lost. It's not just a one-time event; it is an on-going thing escalating over the years. Everyone talks, including me! It's impossible to lipread when we're socializing. Sign works. She is a stay-at-home mother and she has the time to learn if she wants to.

As an adult, using spoken English was Kacie's choice. However, it was no longer Maxel's. Yet as soon as Kacie said, "He's never tried doing anything that is ours," she realized they had been using her language to communicate with each other. Suddenly, there were no words to make amends. Every time he talks with Kacie, Maxel is exhausted from time-consuming and numerous repetitions to correct misunderstandings. He is telling her: "I have a solution to our communication difficulties and you are not interested!" Having different expectations about which language to use escalated their conflict. Kacie is comfortable communicating in spoken English, whereas Maxel finds ASL more effective. Another layer was the disagreement over priorities about making time for communication. Kacie resisted Maxel's dictating her priorities by insisting she spend time learning ASL. However, Maxel does not have the luxury of time for constant missed opportunities for interaction and intimacy with his sibling. Arising from his determination to take advantage of the communication modality he's discovered, ASL, from his perspective Kacie ought to seize the opportunity to use it to move their relationship in a positive direction. This has backfired.

The pitfalls involved in deaf-hearing sibling interactions are quite common and have rarely been discussed openly within families. Even if they identify the breakdowns in communication which are so emotionally charged, non-signing siblings and deaf siblings' bonding becomes further complicated by society's stigma attached to having a deaf sibling, for being a deaf sibling, and for being seen using a language of the hands in public. During the time Maxel and Kacie were growing up, Paul Higgins in *Outsiders in a Hearing World: A Sociology of Deafness* stressed the acceptance of ASL as the bridge to making the DEAF-WORLD more accommodating to those who are non-signing hearing siblings:

> As children and as adults, the members of the deaf community experience frustration and embarrassment, when navigating in a hearing world. However, within the deaf community, easy and "natural" communication is usually taken for granted. In the hearing world it is rarely achieved. Within the deaf community there is no shame in being deaf. Within the hearing world the deaf were often made to feel ashamed until they grew more accustomed to the shaming behavior

of the hearing. The deaf community is, then, partially a response to the unsatisfying interaction which the deaf experience in a hearing world [Higgins 1980, 170].

Was there any inkling that learning ASL and about the DEAF-WORLD would have any positive effect on Kacie and Maxel's relationship? Outsiders are often intrigued with ASL, seeing it as an art form like dance, and often say, "It's beautiful." For Maxel, it has a different meaning. Yet Kacie sees how ASL can make a difference when she offers the suggestion that the next generation might give hope in bringing the siblings closer.

> Yes, if anything positive has come out of it, it's been my awareness, my friends, my family's awareness of the DEAF-WORLD, and sensitivity to it.... I know that some hearing siblings have chosen to embrace their deaf sibling's world and make it their lives, their professions.... My daughter who hears, obviously, hopefully will learn some ASL from him, which I never did; that might be a positive step towards my brother and I having some sort of a relationship.

Even though Kacie is intrigued with the idea of her daughter learning ASL from her brother, Kacie still refuses to acknowledge she is the one who needs ASL to communicate with her brother.

Many hearing siblings have never learned ASL. Warren as an adult saw the possible benefits but fell short of achieving them when he told his sister: "*I know you would have preferred that I were fluent in ASL—that would have been helpful. I did try lessons and later gave up on it. My sense is that would have improved our relationship.*"

Even when siblings mutually agree on the value of learning ASL and being part of the DEAF-WORLD, what other barriers continue to propel non-signing siblings from getting closer to their deaf siblings?

> What I remember most about growing up with a deaf sibling is learning early on to have compassion for individuals with challenges. Most kids are not born with that trait and having a deaf sister taught me empathy at a very early age. Also I was able to witness firsthand other children learning that lesson.

In the above quote, Julie, Marla's sister, knew of many challenges her deaf sister faced interacting with hearing family members including herself. Although her experiences have shaped her sensitivity, she has compartmentalized two perspectives: Her awareness of deaf people's challenges and not learning to sign. Although she expresses compassion as an observer, recognizing ASL is as vital to deaf people as spoken English is to her, in her interactions with her deaf sibling, the invisible curtain of "no ASL" is always present.

She was not alone in her response, even among those who describe their relationship with their deaf sibling as close, like Stefan:

> Let me tell you all something! Unlike Kacie, I have a good relationship with my deaf sister; we spend the holidays together and other family celebrations. We

used our TTYs to stay in touch, but now she prefers using the Video Relay Service (VRS) to call me, using an interpreter, so she can use ASL because she's more expressive using ASL than English. But when we are facing each other, we do just fine. We both know it would have been easier if I knew ASL, but I don't, and we're OK with that. To be honest, I know my sister was always disappointed I didn't learn to sign, I never felt we had to.

Stefan's rationale for never having learned ASL echoes many of the non-signing siblings who were left with a lingering feeling as adults that ASL was a valuable commodity that would add more substance and depth to their sibling bond. Yet, these hearing siblings are frozen in their Oral communication, unable to break the pattern established as children.

David Luterman, a researcher who interviewed hearing teenagers and young adults with deaf siblings, quoted one as saying:

> Robert prefers to sign now and doesn't associate with hearing people if he can help it.... I wish we knew how to sign then and be able to interpret for him so he could understand while the show was on ... he would have been more involved and would have known what was going on. But I realize that is a big issue that probably never will be solved [Luterman and Ross 1991, 52].

Siblings like Stefan and Robert believe it is too late and too complicated to learn ASL. As children, ongoing disputes, histories of bitterness, distrust and stubbornness may have gotten in the way of confronting these beliefs.

Other underlying factors affecting adult siblings' relationships stem from the communication patterns parents use to resolve conflicts among themselves and with their children. These patterns could range from dictatorship style to consensus building. More often than not, siblings' differences about how to communicate are rarely resolved. Instead they pile up in the hope that somehow things will eventually blow over. They don't. Some non-signing siblings, based on their firsthand experiences, later realize the profound and damaging effects of their deaf siblings' exclusion from surrounding chatter and strongly advocated early exposure to ASL for the next generation. Stefan's deaf sister Joy, reminiscing on her childhood, reveals their older sister's recognition of the impact of ASL:

> Yes, I was disappointed but it never bothered me because I thought I was good in lipreading and had good speech. But sometimes, I didn't understand my brother although my siblings understood me. They weren't against me using sign with my friends in front of them but many of my friends' parents were against signing. Now, it is impossible for my siblings to learn to sign. They just can't! But my sister strongly encouraged me to teach her grandchildren ASL. I realized now it was important for them to learn ASL because I missed out on so much in my life.

The urge to reconcile represents a powerful feeling of optimism. If siblings come to an agreement about what they want out of their relationship, they are fortunate if the days, months or years they have left allow them to make up for whatever they lost. Time is neither their enemy nor their friend; it is the accumulation of little things over time that will heal each and therefore, one another.

When non-signing siblings, accustomed to their childhood communication patterns, experience the communication changes set by their deaf siblings, many still feel resistant, resulting in deeper wounds.

> I guess my brother Greg would love to have me to learn to sign; he totally lives in a deaf environment now, and it's where he feels the most comfortable. But when we were growing up, he spoke, and we used lipreading and cued speech. Whenever we spend time together, we communicate just fine. When it's just the two of us, we'll play sports and things where we don't need to talk much. And I do know how to fingerspell. So if he missed lipreading something I say, I spell it and we move on. Like this, for example, I D-O-N-T W-A-N-T T-O B-E H-E-R-E. I'm sure he'd prefer I learn to sign in addition to fingerspelling but it's not a major bone of contention between us, like Kacie has described with her sibling.

The fine thread linking the brothers is Avery's use of fingerspelling and Cued Speech, which function as survival tools anytime speechreading and lipreading break down. Their time together centered on physical activities or games requiring minimal verbal interaction. It would preclude, for example, a heated discussion strategizing about which team might win the Super Bowl. Although Avery supplements his spoken English with fingerspelling rather than learning to sign, their limited communication tools thwart their brotherly bonding, interfering with the natural give-and-take of their interactions. Ongoing dialogues, without communication breakdowns, would bring the siblings a step closer to getting to know one another's opinions, beliefs and reasons behind their thoughts, instead of adopting those of others, like their parents or those in authority positions. As deaf adults matured and immersed themselves in the DEAF-WORLD experiencing everyday interactions, they expressed a yearning for stronger bonds with their hearing siblings, wanting to know more about them as people, as parents, about their jobs; searching for detailed information surrounding their siblings' lives.

Illustrating another barrier to sibling intimacy, one of the non-signers told of a specific misgiving about learning and using ASL. It was almost as if she was at a tipping point that could be a life changer:

> Hmmm. I have a somewhat different perspective. I definitely acknowledge ASL has become an important part of my deaf brother's life but at the same time, it has become a wall between us. I have a feeling if I did learn it, then it would become my responsibility to make sure he knows what's going on and that takes away from me. I think he feels my not learning ASL means I don't love him and ... that's far from the truth. It's nothing personal against him but ... my interests

are elsewhere right now. I do love him and have tried to watch out for him throughout our lives.

Violet, the youngest sibling, was described by her deaf brother, Grant, as the most sensitive one in the family. These two siblings agreed she was his caretaker, a responsibility she took on as a young child. A professor of deaf education, Barbara Luetke-Stahlman, recounts one parent's observations of the siblings' role: "We don't insist that they [the siblings] interpret, but we often discuss how important it is to include Mary Pat in the conversations around her. They are sensitive to her feelings of being left out" (Luetke-Stahlman 1992, 11).

Parents set the expectations for how siblings are to care for one another. Sometimes, children naturally slip into specific roles which parents reward with positive reinforcements. However, unexpected repercussions occur when siblings take on caretaking roles. In Violet's case, Dale Atkins, a psychologist, explains the reasoning behind a caretaker role: "Hearing siblings commonly perceive that they have more responsibilities than their counterparts in caretaking activities for their hearing-impaired sibling.... They worry about giving their hearing-impaired sibling what they are missing, so they interpret for them" (Atkins 1987, 40).

Each time Grant mingles with non-signing hearing relatives or family friends, he is Violet's helpless older brother. As much as he appreciates Violet's efforts to include him, knowing she tried her best, he says it just never works: "*I felt I am not important, brushed aside, off in a corner. Once in a while my sister would look at me and point out which relative was talking and try to summarize the conversation, but they'd forget to include me.*"

The drama between siblings like Grant and Violet continues over many years, building a wall between them. As time passes and siblings' roles evolve from caring for someone to being cared for, their unresolved tensions get thicker. The issue isn't just between the siblings; it becomes the entire family's issue. Their interaction has consequences: Violet was astute enough to recognize if she had been the *only* family member who knew ASL, her chances of being trapped with expanding her caretaking role would be greater. Non-signing family members and her deaf brother would come to expect her to facilitate their interactions. Involving the non-signing family members in discussions surrounding communication access could potentially ease the tensions between the siblings.

In retrospect, when deaf siblings described their non-signing hearing siblings' efforts to reduce their isolation, they saw potential allies anticipating they would become close. However, Enid, one of the non-signing siblings, expressed her increased despair at her sister's finding an ally outside of the family:

I'm with you, Violet! I haven't learned ASL though I've met people who've seemed to pick it up so easily, I'm green with envy! I too have worked hard to include my sister by trying to tell her what people have said and have nagged my siblings to include her, and much as I'd love to know ASL, I can't seem to find the time to do it. Even hanging out with her and her friends hasn't motivated me to pursue it. I know she wants me to learn it; it's connected with respect for her and her language, but I haven't figured out how to fit it into my busy life what with family and work commitments. And I do think ASL is a beautiful language. My sister considers her deaf friends to be her family, whereas we, her blood family, are second rate because we don't know or use ASL.

The ramifications of the deaf siblings searching for intimate relationships outside of the family have a tremendous effect on deaf and hearing siblings' well-being. There is juxtaposition: I am included yet I am also excluded. Deaf siblings find deaf peers in the DEAF-WORLD as natural substitutes for developing close relationships. However, by doing so, they increase the risk that they will be apathetic towards getting closer to their sibling.

Hearing siblings feel the sting of the deaf sibling's rejection, but Enid's deaf sister Micki defends ASL as her lifeline: "*Yes, I do struggle to understand my hearing siblings. When they make the effort to talk to me, I nod, pretending to understand but I'm nodding while grasping bits here and there, guessing what they're saying, often asking them to repeat.*"

Some siblings perceive learning ASL as a tool they chose not to use. However, Risa's younger sister, an ASL interpreter, was the inspiration for giving her a brother she longed for:

> I learned to Sign after I left home. During our growing up years, my brother and I struggled with speech and lipreading. I know it stifled and inhibited our interactions. After I learned to Sign, I was able to develop a close and comfortable relationship with my brother. Sign puts us on an equal footing where theoretically neither of us has to struggle. Although I have to admit since ASL is a second language for me, I'm always struggling to express myself in it, but I think less than he would be struggling to lipread me.

As siblings like Risa who saw ASL as a necessity for building a relationship with her deaf brother, deaf and hearing siblings have the power to let go of their past and recognize they do not have to live by their childhood histories and patterns.

Since ASL and the DEAF-WORLD are inseparable, French linguist Francois Grosjean highlights the kinship:

> Both as an instrument of communication and as a symbol of group identity, language is accompanied by attitudes and values held by its users and also by persons who do not know the language. For example, although few readers of this book know American Sign Language, most hold some value judgment about this manual-visual language, which they may have seen on TV. What is important to

realize, however, is that attitudes toward a language—whether it is beautiful, efficient, rich and so on—are often confounded with attitudes toward the language from attitudes toward its users, the Deaf [Grosjean 1982, 117].

Risa's willingness to seek change required taking small steps to have a closer relationship with her deaf brother. To her, it was worth the time invested and the continued effort necessary to learn ASL, in spite of the tedious task of memorizing vocabulary and using the grammar unlike hers. During the interview, her brother expressed his support, "*She was nervous. She would gesture to make sure I understood. I told her she was good and saw that she was relieved.*" Deaf siblings were in agreement that ASL was the bridge to getting closer to their siblings, and they had come to that conclusion not only based on their interactions in ASL with their peers, but the *opportunity* to have a closer relationship with their sibling made it even more compelling. Nevertheless, with Risa as the exception, all of the non-signing siblings, who used spoken English with their deaf siblings as children, continued to follow their parents' communication model. With these unresolved differences, these siblings remained unsatisfied in their relationships.

Parents are the decision-makers; they decide what language will be used in the rearing of their deaf child. They model what professionals advise them to do, often tempered with their own experiences and beliefs. The agony of having a deaf child did not prevent one sibling's mother from bringing her judgment to the advice of professionals. Randall was grateful for his mother's defined goal: communicating with her deaf child now!

When she found out I was deaf, she asked the doctor, "What should I do?" She was lucky the doctor recommended she explore different methods such as oralism, Cued Speech, and others. My mom visited an oral school and observed there briefly. With Cued Speech programs, it was difficult because mom had to call different places and most of them were located too far since she preferred a program closer to home. Then, she went to Parkland school.[1] She said what impressed her mostly was when she went there ... a teacher had a ball and when she signed "ball," I copied it right away. Mom was taken aback and asked what the sign meant. She was blown away by how quickly I was able to grasp the idea. Mom wanted to also check out the Clarke School for the Deaf. She said what was most convincing, which led her decision not to use the Oral approach, was when they advised her: "You'd have to wait between two to three years where you cannot communicate with your son. Then, it will be fine afterward." They quickly added that she couldn't sign either; the focus was to be solely based on speech. Mom asked herself whether she could bear two years during a dinner meal not communicating at all with me.

The hearing mother wanted her deaf child to have what her son and every child has when acquiring language: a mother tongue, which provides access to one another's conversations and reinforces the power of "learning by osmosis."

One of the deaf siblings, Rami, gave an example of the osmosis effect pervading the interaction between a hearing mother and her seven-year-old deaf daughter:

> There was a family of three—the mother was a fluent signer—an interpreter quality. The father signed too but had mediocre skills. Approximately two weeks after having found out about their kid's hearing, the mother registered for a sign class. She was in a conversation with another hearing mother. They were talking, not signing, with one another. As soon as she turned and saw her kid approaching, she automatically switched to signing so that her daughter could watch their conversation. The other mother caught on and started signing too. The kid watched their conversation for a while—that is learning by osmosis. Then, the kid would ask the mother a question; the mother would teach the kid by signing, "When you tap me, please say excuse me" so the kid would sign, "Excuse me" and the mother would turn to the other mother and say, "Excuse me" to proceed with her conversation with her daughter. They would converse in ASL and the mother would answer her daughter's question. If the daughter didn't understand, she would ask her mother to fingerspell again. The mother adapted the fingerspelling by using another communication mode, cued-speech, so that way the kid would perfectly pronounce the word she missed. Then, the mother would use ASL to sign the meaning of the word. Then, they proceeded with the rest of the conversation. This girl was profoundly deaf and was capable of speaking, signing and learning simultaneously from the conversations she was observing and understanding.

Unequivocally a person needs to have effective and accessible communication at an early age in order to develop language. "Parents and siblings need to put forth all effort they can to make sure the communication environment is visually accessible, not only when addressing the deaf child. Seeing how adults talk to each other is one of the major ways that children learn how people communicate, negotiate, and share" (Marschark and Hauser 2012, 62). Furthermore, to be a functional member of American society, all children need to be literate and communicate naturally, receptively and expressively.

How is it that neurologically normal persons like the deaf people Pinker describes are made to feel so diminished based solely on hearing status, not intelligence, talents or ability to interact with people? Why was being deaf so stigmatized? What the policy makers gain by stigmatizing deaf people was not only power over deaf education but the financial gains to be had from jobs as a result of the consequences of Oralism: a century of dismal educational achievement leading to severe unemployment and underemployment of several generations of deaf people who, unlike their deaf predecessors prior to 1880, rarely achieved literacy. In 1996, three scholars, Harlan Lane, Robert Hoffmeister and Ben Bahan, reported the profound consequences: "We have seen that, after nearly a century of Oralism, the average Deaf high school graduate had achieved a third-grade education. Alas, after twenty-five years of TC, the results have not improved" (Lane and Hoffmeister and Bahan 1996, 271). Each generation strives to do better than the previous generation in the field of education through hands-on approaches with teaching, training, and research. The third-grade reading level among deaf children had become the norm using the English-based Sign systems lacking the fundamentals of a language.

Simultaneously, ASL had begun to earn respect in academic circles, prompting educators to search for a different approach. Deaf professionals, strong proponents of language acquisition in the field of deaf education, fought to use bilingual techniques with deaf children. An exemplary approach was taken by a native ASL user from a deaf family, Marie Phillips, who pioneered in the Bicultural Bilingual (Bi-Bi) approach, believing that deaf children could become bilingual, acquiring ASL and English simultaneously. She took the lead as the Bilingual-Bicultural Coordinator of the Learning Center for the Deaf in Framingham, Massachusetts, creating an academic environment where deaf children would become bilingual, equally proficient in ASL and English (The Learning Center for the Deaf n.d.). Few deaf schools sought to use her model by sending their educators to observe and get trained using her approach for research. The majority of professionals and families remained skeptical about the long-held belief that learning ASL inhibits learning speech. The evidence proved otherwise, as one educator, Dr. Mark Marschark, declared:

> It is easy enough to understand the desire of most hearing parents to have a child who speaks and acts normally. The truth is, however, that most deaf children will never sound like their hearing brothers and sisters. Delaying the learning of sign language in the hope of developing better speaking skills in deaf children simply does not work in most cases. In fact, such delays can make matters more difficult for both children and their parents. The first years of life are when basic language skills develop, and the first two to three years are generally recognized as a critical period for language learning. There is no substitute for natural language learning, and language acquisition that begins at age three or four is not natural [M. Marschark 1997, 14–15].

In addition, although the elementary and middle schools on the campus of Gallaudet University provided a Bi-Bi program through the groundbreaking efforts of M.J. Bienvenu, Professor of ASL and Deaf studies, none of the siblings in this study attended Bi-Bi programs. However, the parents who sent their deaf children to the few Bi-Bi schools are indications that respect for using ASL had arrived, at least in some families.

As they told their stories, the siblings we interviewed searched for tools to alleviate the emotional scars resulting from their parents' continued use of only speech and lipreading to communicate with their deaf family member. For some, the psychological reverberations created an impenetrable distance between deaf and hearing siblings. For others, like a magnet the search brought them together, conveyed to us in soul-searching stories, often defining their sibling relationships on a continuum—from best friends to bitter enemies. The consequent lack of access to a shared language ostracized some deaf siblings who never felt at home in their families. Regardless of constant pleas by parents and hearing siblings insisting deaf siblings be at home for family gatherings, many deaf siblings ultimately substituted deaf peers for family. The bond these deaf siblings had with their peers was too powerful to ignore: The shared deaf identity and a common language—ASL—and their cultural ties, created a world in which they felt at home. Even when families are using sign and spoken English in the home, creating the experience of bilingualism, home is often the place where biculturalism—deaf culture—is absent. Being bilingual does not guarantee biculturalism. By immersing the family in deaf community events, they learn the social rules and ways to interact in the DEAF-WORLD, similar to living in a foreign country, which is traditionally been the way to absorb that country's culture.

Paddy Ladd, a British deaf scholar of *Understanding Deaf Culture: In Search of Deafhood*, poses the following question:

> Imagine that all children with a hearing loss on a scale that inhibits meaningful interactions with mainstream societies were brought up bilingually and biculturally; that they were told throughout their childhood, "By learning both spoken and sign languages, you can learn to navigate your life path in and around two cultures and two communities, selecting whatever you wish for from either in order to build your own lives." Is this not culturally-centered perspective a more healthy social philosophy than the medical one which stresses the shamefulness of association with signing communities? [Ladd 2003, 34].

The shamefulness of association with signing communities is a form of oppression of deaf people and their families, especially their siblings.

One hearing sibling, Anita, who worked as an educational interpreter for deaf students, shared her concerns:

> There was this condescending attitude towards these deaf kids who were treated as dummies because they didn't know a lot of things. Yet, on the other hand, they didn't want you to use ASL, they wanted you to Sign in English. The woman who was running the department couldn't really Sign very well and she was "running" the department! Additionally, they didn't treat these kids as though they were part of the mainstream. They had to come to a special resource room for us to tutor them and they were seen as different. The staff knew that there were those types of people working there, but they all backed down. None of them would get into those people's faces. They were afraid.

This was yet another instance of the lingering effects of Milan, over one hundred years later, when MCE systems were used. As a sibling of a deaf person and an ASL interpreter, she was baffled at administrators' decision to forbid ASL, thereby rejecting deaf culture and deaf people; she had seen ASL not only open her deaf brother's mind, but ASL was the link to his understanding of the world around him. Perhaps most critical, she was working in an educational system that diminished and inhibited deaf children's psychological and cognitive development. When she saw how engaged she and her brother could be casually chatting in ASL about evolution, it was an epiphany. No longer were their conversations limited to three- or four-word question-and-answer sentences like what they did when he was in an oral elementary school. As soon as her brother transferred to the state residential deaf school, she witnessed his cognitive, linguistic, and cultural competency flourishing with his classmates and deaf house-parents and then, at home, with her. Consequently, she adopted a worldview about the presence of ASL as the *vehicle* for her and her deaf brother to interact as equals.

Transformations Toward Equality

While the events of the late twentieth and early twenty-first century caused an upheaval in the education of deaf children and within their families, simultaneously, earthquakes occurred in the microcosm of the DEAF-WORLD: Gallaudet University, the world's only institution of higher education for deaf and hard of hearing, deaf-blind, and late-deafened students. In 1988, the Board of Trustees appointed a hearing person as the incoming president. To protest, three deaf representatives met with the Board Chair, Dr. Jane Bassett Spilman: "It was at this meeting Spilman is purported to have said, 'Deaf people are not ready to function in a hearing world,' a statement she later said was misinterpreted. She had used a double negative" (Gannon 2002, 37).

Nevertheless, student protests erupted, headlined with banners of "Deaf President Now (DPN)." Protesters were supported not only by faculty members but also by Gallaudet alumni and local communities throughout the country, causing a campus shutdown, reminiscent of student protests during the 1960s Civil Rights movement. The Board finally relented, appointing I. King Jordan, a late-deafened candidate, to the position. Choosing a late-deafened person, rather than several congenitally deaf candidates, was a compromise giving a message to the world: a person with a hearing loss was now acceptable and capable of leading. The tensions between students and faculty with the board caused more than a ripple effect throughout the country, raising awareness that being deaf was a *prerequisite* for the incoming president of Gallaudet University. Siblings we interviewed were aware of the DPN events at Gallaudet, though the younger ones learned about it as history at DEAF-WORLD lectures about the far-reaching effects of audism. The siblings' stories unmasked how audism permeated their homes and school environment and have continued to create further emotional and social distancing from their families and peers.

Additionally, even within the core of the DEAF-WORLD, different forms of audism existed. The most prominent example was the 2006 protest surrounding the appointment of Dr. Jane Fernandes as the next president of Gallaudet University. However, shades of audism were present long before, when she was the provost responsible for the development of the Strategic Plan for Gallaudet's future. As a deaf woman in a powerful leadership position at the world's only deaf university, she never took advantage of the opportunity to take a stand to define the university's language policy as one that gave equal value and equal respect to ASL and English. Instead she created a division, forcing students and faculty to support her values for inclusion, surrounding deaf people's lives with all forms of MCE communication systems at the expense of ASL, and perpetuating Gallaudet's long-term policy that neither faculty nor students needed to attain fluency in ASL, a blatant form of audism (Bauman, "Postscript: Gallaudet Protests of 2006 and the Myths of In/Exclusion" 2008).

Internal and long-held beliefs about ASL by the families we interviewed are nearly impossible to ignore. Why should deaf siblings continue to enable the oppressive behaviors and attitudes by both deaf and hearing people? Like other minority cultures, most deaf people weren't given a chance to develop their own identities without any filters, similar to Native Americans who were taken from reservations and placed in white families. Unaware of the effects audism may have on them, deaf people are likely to oppress one another. The acceptance of audist behaviors may be explained by a theory called dysconscious audism, as proposed by Genie Gertz:

> [A] sizable group of Deaf people who would be categorized as "dysconscious audists" because they haven't developed their own Deaf consciousness and identity to the fullest. Generally their Deaf consciousness is distorted to varying degrees. Dysconscious audistic Deaf people unwittingly help to continue the kind of victimized thinking that they are responsible for their failure. Such thinking enables hearing people to continue pathologizing Deaf people [Gertz 2008, 222–223].

Audist behavior may be subtle, especially if deaf people perceive themselves as not whole. Deaf people's varied responses to oppression are inconsistent. Dr. Gertz expands the subtlety of oppression by stating the differences in the awareness a person has toward audist behavior:

> The marked difference between "unconscious" and "dysconscious" when used with the word audism is that the word unconscious implies that the person is

completely unaware whereas the word dysconscious implies that the person does have an inkling of his or her consciousness but does not yet realize it is impaired. Some Deaf individuals choose to do nothing about it or to take a "so be it" attitude. In this manner, it is not that they are completely unaware of the issues; it's just their decision on how to live with them [Gertz 2008, 223].

Why is it so painful that many barely think about it, just adapt and get on with their lives, doing what it takes to survive daily doses of oppression? Rose Pizzo, in her memoir *Growing Up Deaf: Issues of Communication in a Hearing World,* described her awakening:

> I remember feeling I didn't know what was going on but I didn't think anything was wrong. I thought I was normal not to understand. That was just part of my life. I just didn't understand and I thought it was O.K. I didn't realize it was not O.K. until I married Vincent. I was so excited. Vincent and I could sign with each other, in our own home. My whole life, while I was growing up, I had to be with hearing people. Finally, in my house, my home, I could communicate easily with my husband, morning, noon and night, twenty-four hours a day. Wow [Pizzo 2001, 124]!

We have noted how the series of events shaped the varied identities and communication modalities of the siblings we met. In the meantime, their hearing siblings, like Marla's brother Joseph, experience the emotional backlashes since siblings typically are mutually dependent on one another.

> I saw a big change at some point in her life—when I perceived her as being angry at the world for trying to assimilate her into the hearing world. The notion of a deaf world and hearing world being completely different and at odds with each other seemed sad to me. We are rather distant so I don't know, yet I suspect some of this thinking still exists today.

The anger is never understood because siblings have yet to find common ground and often don't know why they are at odds. The assumption is if one sibling changes, then it means the change is an attack on the other siblings when the change is really about finding one's place in the family and even the world.

Some deaf and hearing siblings grew up believing that being deaf and using sign was something to be ashamed of; others grew up with a strong sense of pride in themselves or their deaf siblings as deaf people, respecting ASL and deaf culture. Several hearing siblings struggled to comprehend the pride, unable to identify or feel connected to their deaf siblings' DEAF-WORLD. In families, where siblings are taught "doing kindness unto others" as a way of expressing our moral values, there is a feeling of justice to "do the right thing," especially when the caring becomes part of our very being.

Yet situations arise where a sibling's sense of righteousness puts him in such unfamiliar territory—the DEAF-WORLD—that their discomfort takes precedence, even when they respect the culture and feel entitled to be part of it. This was the case when Judy and her siblings were attending an event hosted by their deaf nephew where the majority of guests were deaf adults. To get Larry's attention while he was having a "voice-off" ASL conversation with a friend, even with several attempts to tap on his shoulder and his acknowledgment of her wanting to interrupt, Mary Ann, not knowing ASL, walked away frustrated and impatient, confiding to Judy, "I'll never go to a Deaf event again! It is rude for them to sign and not acknowledge my presence!" This was the very same sibling who, during their childhood, had shown empathy: she defended her deaf brother, kept him in the loop, made the effort to include other deaf people she had run into at bridge games and other social events where hearing individuals predominated. What was familiar to Mary Ann was her comfort in advocating for her brother *in a hearing environment*. However, when it came to the DEAF-WORLD, the reciprocity was naturally expected, yet it wasn't there. As her feelings were kept buried from her brother, behaviors like this contributed to their deteriorating relationship, especially the enormous problem of having to address the language and cultural differences emerging within the family.

Unlike their hearing siblings, like Mary Ann, who continued to use Oral communication with their deaf siblings, by 2005–2006 when we conducted many of the interviews, some older deaf siblings had personally gone through a transformation. Maxel proudly shared: "*In 1988, the DPN protest happened. My world changed. People said to me before you were the quiet type, now you're protesting.*" Maxel was an active participant in the DPN movement. His transformation, as well as that of other deaf individuals, came not only from the four student leaders of the DPN movement, but also from a group of Gallaudet alumni and deaf professionals known as the "Seven Ducks." They were primarily responsible for the "behind the DPN Movement," along with several key deaf women leaders who maintained an essential relationship with the media, keeping them informed of events as they happened. Many of these leaders, along with numerous others from disability groups, formed coalitions as a result of DPN's getting the press and Congress's attention, that soon after led Congress to pass the Americans with Disabilities Act (ADA) (Office of Communications, Gallaudet University Spring 2013).

The following historical events in the twentieth and twenty-first centuries have transformed the lives of deaf siblings. Consequently, as the century came to an end, their hearing siblings became more aware of the possibilities for more efficient and effective interaction.

Transformational Historical Events

1817+	Establishment of deaf residential schools in USA
1880	Conference of Milan leads to rise of Oralism; banning Sign all over the world; firing deaf teachers; founding of National Association of the Deaf (NAD)
1965	Linguists identified ASL as a language, not broken English
1970+	Deaf people become visible in public theaters, television and movies
1973+	Federal laws promoted deaf children's attendance in mainstream programs including colleges and universities
1988 (and 2006)	Deaf Civil Rights Protests (Deaf President Now) at Gallaudet University
1990	Congress passed the American with Disabilities Act (ADA)
2000+	Technology and Internet access with videophones, pagers, and social media emerge as steps towards functional equivalency

In spite of these events, evidence of progress toward acceptance of deaf people as part of society is far from over and has yet to permeate every family, leaving siblings with much work ahead of them.

Intersectionality

When hearing siblings are with their deaf sibling, oppression often hovers in the background. Sometimes it is in the foreground as well, when engaging with hearing relatives—the vast majority of whom do not know ASL—and during the times hearing siblings would overhear comments about their deaf sibling. Golda described her misgivings about being an ally to her deaf sibling:

> Being an ally to my sister ... I've never said anything and I don't know why. I guess, maybe it's that whole hierarchy. They're my elders and I don't want to say anything. Or maybe I don't think it's worth it. Or maybe it's because my sister's never asked me to, but why should she ask me to? You know, it's like black people are always talking about racism. You need to have white people talking about racism. You need to have hearing people talking to hearing people about audism and oppression. You can't have the deaf person always saying, "You oppressed me." You know, you need to have the hearing person.... So I know ... that I guess, I would be that person.

In order to conquer the premises of audism as a form of oppression, it takes those who are members of the majority culture to confront the issue. Systematic oppression contributes to the complexity of the external influences occurring in society also shaping siblings' identity and position in the family unit.

A black feminist, Patricia Hill Collins, introduced the idea of how various forms of oppression overlap: specifically, intersectionality is "an analysis claiming that systems of race, social class, gender, sexuality, ethnicity, nation, and age form mutually constructing features of social organization" (Collins 2000, 299). Any of these elements may become targets for oppression which are fluid depending on the circumstances. More evidently these forms occur simultaneously where one form of oppression shapes individual's interactions. It begins with the person's internal perception affecting daily relationships. If your brother was raised to think boys are superior to girls, his attitude and behavior towards his female relatives, including his siblings, reinforces the acceptance of these beliefs that eventually become the norm.

Sexual identity and gender roles have also shaped the development of how siblings relate to one another during the socialization process. Sexual identity generally refers to biological differences between males and females; however, there are times at birth when sexual identity is not clearly defined. In addition, in cases where a person "comes out of the closet" or has a sex change, the impact on the sibling relationship is likely to be profound. For example, as siblings mature, they can become more intimate even when unexpected sexuality is revealed:

> AVNA: He was furious that I caused the family uproar when I came out to the family.
> MARLA: What prompted the change in your relationship with your youngest brother?
> AVNA: Well, as kids, we hardly had anything to say to one another. But after the dust settled, we started to chat. We sat down and had great conversations about religion, sexual preference, just about anything. He is more accepting of who I am. I was blunt with him: "I am just telling you I'm a lesbian."

As opposed to the biological perspective, social scientists define gender as culturally imposed masculine, feminine or intersex roles and behaviors. For example, children often challenge their culture's expectations with respect to their talents, intellect, and interests. More specifically, children tend to formulate their own perceptions labeling what the gender role *ought* to be. The symbolic items culturally associated with gender vary in different parts of the world. When family members break gender roles expected within their specific culture, they and their family may be scorned by the community, or worse, by their own relatives. Experts disagree regarding the percentage that biology and the environment each contribute to gender stereotypical behavior. Apparently, evidence supports both; this is the traditional nature-versus-nurture dispute, about the impact of gender roles, decades old (Berger 2008). Marla pinpoints how her earliest memory with gender differences was affected by her youngest brother's birth: *"Joseph, as the only boy, became the joy of the family, especially for my father. It started with the Bris celebration and it ended with Joseph's Bar Mitzvah. Like many cultures including ours, my father had a higher regard for boys and men than for girls and women. And I felt I was being penalized for being female."*

Jasmine reported how her hearing sibling defended her to confront their parents' stereotypes. It is also an example of double oppression from the perspective of a deaf female sibling:

MARLA: Can you explain how your parents were overprotective?
JASMINE: I remember vividly when my sister told me how our parents refused to let her play track and field and when it came to me, she fought them to let me play soccer.
MARLA: Which sister fought for you?
JASMINE: The one who always kept me abreast of family gossip.
MARLA: Why do you think your parents didn't want you to participate in sports?
JASMINE: Of course, I'm deaf and we're girls.

The tentacles of any form of oppression are far-reaching, getting into the person's very soul, regardless of the specific form they take. When deaf people and their hearing families believe deaf people are impaired, implying they need to be fixed, a framing trap is occurring. The trap is set from audist's successful marketing of pathological phrases such as *fix*, *handicapped* and *disabled*, all of which enable victimization mentality. The deaf person then falls into a lifetime spiral of beliefs that they need to be rehabilitated, destroying their independence and self-confidence. Being deaf is as vital to their identity as their gender, sexual orientation or ethnicity, among other identities. The medical model perspective does not recognize or understand this key component of the deaf identity. Kevin described his transformation:

It's hard for me to get this out and to confess ... on the night before Christmas Eve, I did pray to God: "Please make me hearing tomorrow." When I was in high school and during my years at Gallaudet, I looked back thinking how ridiculous that had been and was disgusted with myself for feeling this way. But when I thought about it I realized how normal it had been because my world had changed from when I was mainstreamed, being with the "hearing," having no friends and struggling academically. Somehow I thought it was the ideal normal environment for me. It was how I processed information in my hearing school while not knowing about Gallaudet or a Deaf school. It wasn't until I entered a Deaf school, I found myself totally relieved and in awe with ASL—full access to communication and social interactions. Then, I felt I was normal once again.

The exposure to ASL and a sense of belonging among deaf peers becomes the awakening of self-acceptance. There is an inner peace knowing you're not a person with the disability, but a person with an identity you've created that represents who you are.

The following scenarios are happening in homes throughout the country: The first-born child is hearing. Mom and Dad, who eagerly used Signs, are ecstatic! At nine months old their daughter is Signing to ask for things like "MILK," "MORE," "EAT" or describe her feelings of "COLD" and "HURT." They watch with dismay as their friends struggle to figure out why their non-signing hearing babies are crying or showing signs of temper tantrums. When their best friends' baby arrives and is confirmed deaf, the parents heed the advice of the experts and choose not to sign with their baby, dismissing an effective way to communicate and reduce frustrations. Is it possible that parents don't realize that "a parent's job is rising to the occasion, while the child's job is simply being" (Solomon 2012, 100)? Ironically, it is the parents of the deaf baby who have never heard or wouldn't accept the advice of other experts: "[D]eaf children who receive early exposure to sign communication are more competent in their early language development (and later, reading) than those children who receive only exposure to spoken language" (M. Marschark 1997, 97).

In contrast, primarily in hearing families when speech is valued, is it *not* a form of oppression when the deaf sibling goes to endless hours of speech lessons but hearing siblings do *not* attend ASL classes? How is it possible for a deaf person to learn empathy towards others and lend support, when their thoughts and opinions are often rarely sought or dismissed by hearing siblings' never-ending phrases of "Never mind, it's not important?" What if the oppressor is a sister, uncle, a grandparent or even a deaf brother? One hearing sister, Alma, was concerned about her grandparents' interests: *"All my grandparents can ask is whether or not he can hear and is he going to learn to talk and they look past the fact that my sister is very successful and just fine the way she is."*

Vigilant and Resilient

Several hearing siblings, similar to Alma, perceive their deaf brothers or sisters simply as siblings—people. We all are conscientious, intelligent persons living in the world of scattered sounds. Sounds are everywhere: when we're breathing, among family and friends, our home with its appliances and technological devices, public entities, or even in the silence within us. Nature and its environment with its beauty and melodies were designed just for us. Some sounds are pleasant while others can be a nuisance or even painful. Sometimes we have no control over any of these sounds; we do not take them for granted. If we could put aside what we hear, literally and figuratively in many ways, deaf and hearing siblings do have similar life experiences. We are born, live and die. Deaf and hearing siblings know their lives are similar, yet they are not oblivious to the differences. Are the differences, aside from personalities, interests, and family roles, limited to our hearing status, communication differences, isolation, alienation, among other things, not a part of everyday lives? Before we even identify the factors that either foster or inhibit a deaf and hearing sibling relationship, we must identify the facets encompassed in the deaf experience. Then we will be able to relate to why the intensity of sibling closeness is situated on the continuum from Intimate to Hostile (Cicirelli 1995, Gold 1989).

Deaf siblings inhabit a world where partial information is available; they watch, try to make sense out of what they see, cautiously decide what to do, or simply copy the actions of others. In these vignettes, derived from everyday events, numerous assumptions regarding one another's actions occur, leading to conflicts arising frequently. Each is a sampling of how deaf people confront the sounds surrounding them in different situations:

> Suzanne, sixteen years old, is sitting with her sister Toby at a family gathering, asking her about their upcoming vacation plans. Suddenly Toby's head turns away; cutting off eye contact. Suzanne wondered: "Did someone call Toby's name? Maybe someone fainted or screamed. Did something spill? Is someone laughing or crying so loud that Toby had to see what happened?" Her thoughts went further: "Didn't she realize what she did? She cut me out."

> Wayne, nine years old, is attending a birthday party for Murray, a member of his Little League team. Suddenly he sees the other children heading into another room up the stairs. Wayne follows them, sees pizza on the dinner table and looks for a seat. The only seat left is facing his friend, Sean who is sitting in front of the window. The sun is streaming in behind Sean; Wayne can barely see Sean's face. Does he ask Sean to change seats with him? Would he know enough to ask Murray's mom to lower the shade so he can communicate with his friend? Or does he say nothing and mind his own business?

> Alan, thirty-four years old, eyes glued to his computer screen, turns suddenly to a tap on his shoulder, and has a split second to think about who it might be. He looks up and recognizes a coworker holding an insurance form, needing his signature. He thinks to himself, "I wonder how long she'd been standing there? Did I miss something important she said?"

The deaf adults interviewed shared experiences similar to those of Suzanne, Wayne and Alan, but each had personal cumulative encounters in their sphere inside the hearing world, leading them to devise ways of managing the chaos dominated by sound. These kinds of events force deaf people to be vigilant and resilient, shaping their deaf experience.

At home, deaf siblings have seen how hearing people take sounds for granted. Often hearing siblings are unaware or unfamiliar with subtleties related to sounds shaping their family dynamics; sounds are unpredictable and appear in unanticipated venues. For hearing siblings, sounds bring them closer to the world around them, but Ellen reminisced how sounds have shut her out:

> Ellen's sister, brother and spouses were sitting, hanging out, and chatting the hours away in the living room while Ellen and her deaf husband were sitting by themselves. Ellen was slowly turning the pages of TV Guide, barely looking at them, while Ivan was watching TV.
>
> MARIE: Hey, bro, do you think we should call our cousins and see if we can go over there?
> LESTER: Yeah, why not! Last night, Matt said we could wander over there anytime we want, after dinner.
> MARIE: (on the phone): Hey cousin! We're at home, what's up over there? Oh, great, we'll be there in five minutes!
>
> Suddenly, Ellen noticed the living room was empty. She turned to her husband but he was too preoccupied to even notice. She put down the magazine and rushed into the kitchen.
>
> ELLEN: Mom, where's everyone?
> MOM: They went over to your cousins' house.
> ELLEN: What!? They didn't even ask us to go with them?!?
> MOM: Go! Go! You can go!
> ELLEN: No way! I refuse to! They left us alone here!

Why wasn't Ellen made aware of her siblings' plans? Lester heard the conversation and that was his cue. Happening around her, but beyond her peripheral view, Ellen didn't have the chance to intercept the plan to visit their cousins. The phone call did not foster a shared experience between Ellen and her siblings. Instead it pushed them further apart, unintentionally. The question then becomes: whose responsibility is it to keep isolated family members in the loop?

The deaf experience is only half the equation, marking the deaf sibling's life. What does it have to do with the hearing sibling? Everything. Conversations are a two-way street with siblings actively listening and attentively talking—where each idea is built upon on other ideas, shaping the interaction instead of being stuck in redundancy with constant communication breakdowns. All voices need to be visually present. But this can be difficult when: "The 'voice' of the deaf child is almost always absent, as is that of the former deaf child: the deaf adult. As the deaf adult literally embodies the failed hopes of hearing parents that their child will somehow be transformed into a hearing adult, the deaf adult is a particularly unwelcome participant in seeking a 'solution'" (Wrigley 1996, 123).

What if our siblings chose to have a conversation regarding their respective views on being deaf or hearing, about ASL, isolation, alienation or even about access? Having conversations on these sticky and deeply personal topics will lead siblings to know more about one another's safe places and vulnera-bilities as deaf and hearing people, acknowledging the differences in one another's interactions. Hearing siblings and hearing parents are accustomed to being part of conversations surrounding them, whether actively engaged, eavesdropping, or just observing. Yet in their hearing lives, many remain obliv-ious to parts of conversation gaps that characterize deaf family members' expe-rience. For the majority of deaf people born to hearing parents, the deaf experience almost always begins with a pivotal and life-changing event, similar to Marla's: *"Particularly for the older siblings like me who grew up speaking only, it often took place at Gallaudet, where we felt like we had 'come home.' For the first time, we discovered a place where we saw and finally understood all of the nuances of a conversation: Shades of meaning, humor and sarcasm."*

None of the twenty-two siblings escaped the subtleties of rejection. By the time these siblings had reached adulthood, all had confronted the notion, either at home or from their surroundings, that to be part of the family, sign had to be, whether embraced or rejected. Although deaf children of deaf par-ents who used ASL showed the way for several centuries, there were only a few families exposed to the idea that ASL was guaranteeing fully accessible language acquisition. In a thousand ways, through the beliefs and subsequent actions families took when they rejected ASL, they excluded and deprived deaf siblings of opportunities from reaching their potential to be productive, satisfied, contributing members not only of American society but within their family unit and their sibling relationship.

Marla asked the deaf siblings why they tend to hang out and socialize with deaf people. Each and every one said, *"They're easier to communicate with."* Sheridan echoes their thoughts on the importance of a deaf identity and a communicatively accessible environment:

> [M]any information gaps exist for deaf and hard of hearing children in the process of developing a mature perception of self and identity. If this is true, then it must be addressed at home, in school, and in professional practice with chil-dren who are deaf and hard of hearing. These information gaps can be filled with sensitivity to the impact they can have on a child's growing sense of self, with efforts to create communicatively accessible environments at home and school, through the provision of role models, association with peers, parent and family education programs, and through additions to our curriculum that address these issues for the children [Sheridan 2001, 228].

7

The Fallout

"Her seeing the world as not deaf-friendly was a battle between us. However, I always felt her willingness to defend me meant she loved me."

—Randall

This fictionalized story, "The Funeral," portrays the hostility between deaf and hearing siblings, Zach and Tara, who bring a lifetime of expectations and assumptions about one another to a supercharged event, the death of a loved one. It is not unusual for people to be at their worst, raw with emotions, when death arrives.

The Funeral

"Mom," Tara's voice revealed her exhaustion. "We just got the call from the hospital. She didn't make it. I'll let you know the details about the funeral when Colton and I figure it out, but it'll probably be on Wednesday. Can you let Zach and Violet know? Good. That'll be one less thing I have to do. Thanks."

Thoughts of her brother, Zach, briefly intervened as she hurriedly searched her closets for a black outfit for herself and an appropriate dress for their daughter. "I'm sure he'll be upset. Colton's mom was so fond of him; they had a special bond."

Tara continued to dwell on her mixed feelings towards her brother. "Why is he this way? My friends had older brothers who looked out for them. If anything, Zach has been just the opposite, always taking care of his needs first because he is deaf. I hope we don't have another drama with him at this funeral."

Her thoughts returned to her eulogy. "Will I even find the time to write it?" Her day disappeared, consumed with phone calls. "We're all right. Colton's mom is finally at peace. See you on Wednesday."

When Zach got the news, he immediately called his cousin Brett, using his tty and the relay service (TRS).[1]

Typing his words on his tty: "Hey Brett, did you hear the sad news? GA"

"Yeah, unfortunately I can't make it to the funeral. GA"

"Ah shoot! She was a neat lady! She didn't know sign but she was so patient with me. I need to find an interpreter. Do you know when's the funeral? GA"

"It is the day after tomorrow. Do you think you can find one that fast? GA"

"It is impossible but I've got to try. I have friends who are interpreters. Perhaps teachers of deaf or as last resort, contact an interpreting agency. But I wish you could come! Do you know who else is going? GA"

"Yeah, but Tara hates interpreters. Worst case, I'll bet Tyler will come through for you. GA"

"Remember Tara's wedding a few years ago, when I told Tara I refused to attend if no interpreters were there. She called me a big baby for just asking about getting one or at Uncle Jay's funeral when someone suggested I sit next to mom and lipread her and dad said if I did that I look like I am four years old. Remember that? Anyway, good idea to ask Tyler if I'm stuck. GA"

"You gotta take care of yourself. Hang in there and call me this weekend. GA"

"Sure, will do. Thanks, bye SK SK."

Sadly, he struck out. Wednesday, Tara and her husband's relatives and friends crowded into the funeral home. Zach hugged his sister and her husband, thinking, "I sure hope I can get through this."

He looked around and made sure he had his seat next to his other sister Violet's husband, Tyler, who was ready with pad and pencil. Zach watched and read as Tyler discreetly scribbled notes summarizing the few prayers and the rabbi's brief talk. Then Tara got up and slowly made her way to the podium, placing papers on the lectern.

Zach's heart sank. He could barely look at Tyler's notes. "What! She has a written eulogy! That bitch! She knows it is impossible to lipread from the second row. How dare she not give me her eulogy! I asked and asked for it. I'm her brother. Doesn't that mean anything to her?"

What Zach wants more than anything else is to participate in the shared experience of grieving, to be a member of the community who has lost a loved one. He longs for his family, and especially his siblings, to lend support and to recognize changes need to be made to ensure there is communication access for him. When Zach became a signing person, it challenged his expectations at family gatherings. Since he uses ASL in the deaf community, it was *not* unreasonable for him to expect the same in hearing-dominated events, especially with his family. However, in his eyes, his family barely adapted. Tara, Zach's sister, is oblivious or even hostile to his new expectations. His other sibling's partner, as a newcomer to the family dynamics, was more willing to accommodate: Since no interpreters were available, providing notes was a partial solution.

To his credit, though his efforts were unsuccessful, Zach took responsibility for finding an interpreter. He has learned, through his experiences within the deaf community of ASL users, the presence of an interpreter benefits both hearing and deaf individuals. At the same time, Zach's assumptions about Tara's awareness and sensitivity to his communication needs and what he believed she *ought* to do to meet them resulted in friction. Since he was so consumed with his own needs, it is possible he wasn't able to even consider her priorities. Each sibling is set in their expectations of the other. From Tara's perspective, her resentment escalated over Zach's making a scene about wanting interpreters for family events. She sees it as a deaf issue, thus relieving her from any responsibility or interest that the family might address. Interpreters are not for her but for her brother. She willingly takes care of all details related to the funeral service and burial arrangements, but this item, communication access for her deaf brother, is not even on her radar screen. On the other hand, she is in the midst of grieving herself and perhaps lacked the sensitivity, patience or interest in Zach's needs, especially when she was under so much stress herself. Often at funerals, vulnerabilities become visible. As a result, siblings tend to lend support to one another. In this case, neither Zach nor Tara had the empathy to set aside their tensions, partially because expectations were not clearly communicated or acknowledged.

In attempts to survive isolation, deaf siblings yearn to lean on their first natural playmates and peers, hearing siblings, rather than their parents as preferred allies to ameliorate isolation. Unrelenting isolation is fundamental to the deaf experience. Throughout the interviews all of the deaf siblings elaborated on their isolation at home or at extended family gatherings. Even those deaf siblings whose parents or sibling used sign continued to experience isolation, especially at mealtimes. Isolation meant not having access to both meaningful *and* trivial family conversations. They missed tidbits about relatives, information about upcoming events, jokes, stories of family histories or arguments, all revealing nuances of family dynamics. They described their deprivation of these everyday conversations—the interactions of chatter—the critical building blocks of human relationships. As a response to isolation, most deaf siblings believed a common language with their hearing sibling was the absolute answer. Embedded in their thinking was: My hearing sibling is quite capable of using facial expressions, body language, and hand-signals which are all the components of the visual-gestural language, ASL. If I use ASL, why doesn't my hearing sibling use ASL too? On the other side of the same conversation, Ashley was not alone in stating this: *"We read lips ... she reads lips very well. That's basically the way we have communicated with her at home ... and it works. Of course, she's also fluent in sign."* Regardless of the language usage, both deaf and hearing siblings recognize using the same language was fundamental for effective communication. However, for deaf siblings, there is an underlying trauma being overlooked. Is it normal not to understand chatting relatives, parents arguing, mealtime discussions, or plans about your sibling's after-school activities? Several deaf siblings grew up with this belief. They accepted it as the hearing world, their sibling's territory, and had no expectations or awareness that they were *entitled* to it themselves. Deaf siblings settled for the hearing sibling's lack of action to include them in these daily dialogues as part of everyday experience. On the other hand, some deaf siblings grew up believing family members were people they could rely on for support. They pursued their hearing sibling to collude with them in combating isolation. When a sister or brother didn't act accordingly, deaf siblings became aware of their own resentment.

In 1913, George Veditz, deaf president of National Association of the Deaf (NAD), launched a film, *The Preservation of Sign Language*, at the NAD conference as a response to the devastating aftermath of the 1880 Conference of Milan. For decades he left his mark: "As long as we have deaf people on earth we will have signs.... It is my hope that we will all love and guard our beautiful sign language as the noblest gift God has given to deaf people" (Padden and Humphrey 1988, 36). In 2010—almost a century after George Veditz's important historical film—the International Council on Education of the Deaf rescinded the edict of the 1880 Milan Conference.[2] The deaf siblings we interviewed, like deaf people worldwide, seek other deaf people or hearing people who use ASL, as friends or partners. Shared identity and fascination with sign is the magnet drawing deaf people together regardless of whether they use oral communication, MCE or other forms of communication systems such as Cued Speech. As a minority in a hearing society, even for those who were raised by deaf parents, isolation is an inescapable part of their lives. As a result of having found the DEAF-WORLD, their resiliency was not only tested but shaken. Each deaf interviewee confessed it was an emotional experience filling a void. Their response to the DEAF-WORLD shaped not only their own identities but future interactions with hearing people, even with immediate family members. Some reacted bitterly about what they had missed growing up and shared their anger intimately with deaf friends. Others became depressed and either demanded or pleaded with family members to sign. Several accepted that their parents and siblings did the best they could with the advice received from professionals, and made peace with the reality that the family was not likely to change. Others settled for the status quo but kept trying to find ways to expose siblings (and other family members) to the DEAF-WORLD, with the expectation these non-signers would be willing to join it, by learning ASL.

With one exception, the hearing siblings who used speech and lipreading as children with their deaf siblings continued to do as adults. As children, they viewed these conversations as part of their daily lives. In retrospect, every adult non-signing hearing sibling admitted remorse. All wished they had learned sign and were convinced that the relationship with their deaf siblings would be different, if not better, if they had. Ashley revealed ambivalent feelings when she said, "*I just feel like I should be able to talk to her in whatever way she would like.*" But oral communication was all they knew. These hearing siblings admitted lipreading and speech were neither adequate nor satisfying in their adult lives, but having no other tools, they settled by believing it must have worked, tolerating the concomitant strain it put on adult face-to-face interactions with their deaf siblings. Complacency came from infrequent contact with one another as adults.

For much of these siblings' growing up years, deaf siblings learned to tolerate these impediments; it was all they knew, too. Oral communication as a common language had major hurdles, which they explicitly defined. Constant interruptions to clarify misunderstandings or missed words and phrases were a nuisance. Endless repetitions with guesswork for words neither one could understand, or long pauses to allow for rephrasing and winging it while groping for alternative ways to say something simpler. Using spoken English made what should have been a simple conversation, if the barriers weren't there, stressful and exhausting. Isolation becomes the trigger for a multitude of emotions interfering with both deaf and hearing people's lives. Deaf siblings' stories revealed how families constantly made decisions without their input, thus depriving them of opportunities to negotiate their thoughts, opinions, or interests about everyday events. Increasing emotional distance, families often made assumptions about the deaf sibling's preferences, with no consideration for their evolving tastes or desires. Deaf siblings would see their hearing sibling arguing with their parents about something, then be told, "Let's go. Why aren't you ready?" There was no room for discussion or understanding what had just happened, that lead to the argument in the first place. Daily instances like these showed deaf siblings had little or no control of their lives that might have led to emotional consequences: depression. Deaf siblings began to believe: "I am invalid. My sister always knows more than me." These never-ending experiences gnawed at the sibling connection.

The "sin of omission" is an intentional behavior, but the person is often not aware that it is a power play. Other disciplines have looked at how the power directed at others comes from within and reverberates within families. Foucault introduces the concept of power as a form of resistance which is a positive response to restrictions (Foucault 1994). When hearing family members receive and fail to share what they've learned through radio, idle chatter, or overhearing conversations, how do their deaf siblings respond? It depends on how their power of resistance is used: Many will not be able to respond since they do not know they've missed anything. Others may have seen something happening, but keep it to themselves for fear of appearing stupid, intrusive, or a pest. The repercussions, however, may extend far beyond the family experience to what could be life-threatening events such as unawareness of weather-related warnings or last-minute announcements on loudspeakers in airports or bus stations. With today's technology, deaf individuals have the potential to use the power of resistance they already have within themselves to pursue visual printed information, in the case of captioning, texting, or digital message boards in public places.

Anger and jealousy arise because siblings naturally have certain expectations of one another. Sometimes they are met but disappointments are inevitable, leading to resentment. So much time and energy are expended trying to impose one's expectations, the anguish involved hurts both siblings and tends to tarnish fragile sibling bonds. In a family setting it is difficult for deaf people to predict whether their sibling will sign or orally summarize what others are saying or even tell them whether someone is talking *to* them. Although many deaf siblings were appreciative of their siblings' willingness to provide access, at the same time, the power imbalance—with the hearing sibling holding the reins—had the potential to negatively affect the relationship because it felt like a violation of trust, when no meta-conversations were conducted about it. Imagine being at the mercy of your sibling to keep you in the loop: If your hearing brother is in a bad mood because his team just lost the pennant, you're out of luck. Or maybe you just had a huge argument over whose turn it was to take out the garbage, and your sister's face suddenly turned pale. She overheard mom and dad arguing and both of you felt the door slam as dad walked out. Will she tell you what just happened? Uncertainty left deaf siblings in a constant emotional state of anxiety, interfering with their ability to negotiate access. However, once they experienced the ease of give-and-take of ASL with deaf peers, it became more difficult for them to accept the status quo of superficial oral communication at home. The striking differences were an awakening, leading several to realize perhaps they would never achieve the same level of intimacy with their own family members they had with their deaf family, especially with hearing siblings. For these deaf siblings, speech and lipreading were not considered a common language and did nothing to alleviate isolation. Instead, it pushed them towards the edge, isolating them further.

Children Learn What They Live

Hearing siblings witnessed isolation leaving its mark. The twelve hearing siblings we interviewed were aware, though in differing degrees, that their deaf siblings were left out of family exchanges and banter. Typically, the family might be sitting at the dinner table. Everyone was participating in or overhearing family conversations, but deaf siblings were there too, invisibly staring into space, possibly exhausted from chasing conversations. The young hearing children, bewildered by their deaf sibling's exclusion, were unsure whether or not anyone saw what they saw. Not knowing what to do or what to make of their uneasiness, they kept it to themselves. Confusion spilled into feelings towards their parents, as the hearing siblings found themselves bombarded with many unanswered questions: "Why am I an integral part of these daily conversations but my parents and siblings constantly exclude my brother? What is this gnawing pain in my stomach? What am I supposed to do?" Yet the hearing siblings all went on with their busy lives. As adults, they found their own way to maneuver around these issues. Their level of awareness was on a continuum, with behavior revealing the extent of actions taken to provide access for their deaf siblings at home, with relatives at family gatherings or with friends and strangers. Several siblings barely noticed their deaf sister or brother's isolation, taking little or no action. Others accepted the isolation as the deaf sibling's life journey, which had nothing to do with theirs, or saw it but did not want to take on the obligation of keeping their sibling in the loop. In contrast, some hearing siblings conquered confusion by taking action to stop the isolation. Perhaps others carried unresolved bewilderment into their adult lives.

As adults, some hearing siblings continued having intimate relationships with relatives and noticed their deaf siblings not chatting with grandma or a favorite uncle, but sitting in a corner reading. Deaf siblings missing innumerable opportunities to connect with hearing relatives pained several hearing siblings. Simultaneously, several hearing siblings who became involved in the DEAF-WORLD believed the relatives were deprived of the chance to learn about a rich, diverse, interesting culture from the perspective of a deaf person. From a multitude of gatherings where the isolation occurred, the deaf and hearing siblings heard the family's message: the deaf siblings were not equal family members.

NEVER MIND. IT'S NOT IMPORTANT.

JUDY: These phrases sure push my buttons and I know they push my deaf brother's buttons too. I can remember my brother saying, "If you said it, then let me decide whether or not it is important." And my sister would fill him in!

MARLA: I never knew what to expect. Depending on her mood, Julie would fill me in but too often I saw these words: "Never Mind, It is not Important." Every time she rolled her eyes, my stomach would start to churn. Yet I knew we both hated the isolation ... couldn't we just deal with it?

Over a span of many centuries, historical events and cultural beliefs have had a profound impact on the cognitive, emotional and social well-being of deaf people. Whereas isolation is cruel to the soul as it creeps up unexpectedly, helplessness is the true silent killer; it annihilates opportunities for families to bond. Every time a parent or a sibling says words reflecting the nuances of, "Never mind, it's not important," they are depriving the child (or sibling) of getting to know one another. It may seem trivial, but each time it happens, each is deprived of the information necessary to know about one another's interests, habits, opinions, values and beliefs. Daily conversations allow individuals to build relationships. "Never mind. It's not important," implies "I don't want to take the time to have a relationship with you."

Family bonding evolves over a lifetime of experiences with parents, siblings and relatives. All siblings compare themselves to one another and carefully scrutinize how they are treated in the family by parents and relatives, but in the case of deaf and hearing siblings, there is additional complexity. Survival mechanisms took over so that deaf siblings could deal with isolation, even though they lead to self-deprecating thoughts. For example, the deaf siblings saw the hearing sibling laughing but missed the words preceding the laughter. Feeling anxious, deaf siblings began to wonder, "What's going on? What are they laughing about? I wish I knew. Why couldn't I laugh too?" Despite attempts to engage hearing siblings as allies to avoid isolation, all the deaf siblings from hearing families wondered, "What about me? Do I matter?" Like their hearing siblings, deaf siblings accepted the message they saw repeatedly: "Family is important ... you are part of the family," but the deaf siblings were perturbed and taunted by a lifetime of conflicting family messages: "We want you to come for Thanksgiving," but when they arrived, they became invisible and isolated. Fluttering lips ping-ponging back and forth were impossible to follow. As they tried, in vain, to keep up with the conversations, self-esteem was shattered. How could they reveal who *they* were—their likes, dislikes, knowledge, interests, skills or opinions? While admiring the conversations as belonging to their family members, deaf siblings' contributions have been minimal. Is it possible to live by the illusions of others, totally unaware of one's own? As mere bystanders instead of as participants, deaf family members had intense emotions that predictably spilled into relationships with sisters or brothers who, by virtue of being hearing, contributed to their isolation in spite of many well-intentioned attempts to prevent or forestall it.

Counter to the biopower and resistance power that were applied to sibling relationships, Foucault presents *Power as Productive* as a means to discover power by reframing perceptions of the obstacles (Foucault 1994). Tackling the inner voice while engaging in dialogue with others, leads to the realization that power actually exists within each of us, though we may not have acknowledged or asserted it yet. It can be a catalyst for change, by seeking ways to engage in dialogue and take a stand regarding obstacles deaf and hearing siblings encounter in their everyday lives as they interact with one another and with non-signers. As they navigate, each experience unravels their place in the world. The most pervasive obstruction is that the dominant language in America is not ASL. Spoken English is everywhere: in hearing families, neighborhoods, schools, hospitals and public events. Imagine a dinner invitation hosted by a hearing non-signing sibling who invites not only the deaf sibling but two non-signing families to join them. Lipreading and using speech to chase conversations is the norm for most deaf siblings. While hearing and deaf siblings agree that engaging in conversations one-on-one *may* work, when more than two people are involved, equal participation fails. Deaf individuals are surrounded by social norms—created, established, and adopted by those who hear. It may be common to invite relatives when a family member visits from out of town. Even if the host informs the deaf sibling of other relatives joining for dinner, is there communication between them about how that decision and its consequences of inevitable breakdowns was made in the first place? What options can they use to address the communication access issue surrounding three or more people involved in conversations? Some potential solutions may include scarce funds which ultimately will have aftereffects forcing unexpected change in people's lives: paying for ASL classes, hiring ASL interpreters, or taking advantage of technical accessibility services. Daily occurrences where these obstacles—dominant language, social norms, decision-makers and how money is allocated—emerge simultaneously in a variety of settings have the capacity to paralyze deaf and hearing siblings. By surrendering and relinquishing their potential for empowerment, they stagnate on their unequal playing fields.

Non-signing hearing siblings can choose to stay in their hearing world and not be affected by these obstacles. But deaf siblings and signing hearing siblings, who spend most of their time bumping into these obstacles, cannot escape. Affirmative statements such as "I am as entitled as they are to enjoy mingling with family and relatives," or "We are all in this together where no one deserves to be excluded in our family," are stepping stones to making a significant change within ourselves and other fellow deaf and hearing siblings. *Productive power,* through ongoing colloquy, stimulates us to respect ourselves as we engage in self-advocacy, become empowered and ultimately fight for justice.

8

Magnet Secrets

"Just as I was leaving for the prom, my older deaf brother appeared with a baseball bat, ready to protect me."—Shannon

This section will disclose uncharted territory and unique findings, rarely mentioned by other researchers, about how deaf and hearing siblings interact with one another during the years their adult relationship is evolving. Both deaf and hearing siblings went into detail, particularly about the behaviors of the hearing sibling aimed at alleviating their deaf sibling's isolation. The deaf siblings' reactions to what hearing siblings did were deeply entwined with the development of the hearing siblings' behaviors, like the two sides of a coin at diametrically opposite ends and everything in between. By virtue of our mutual experiences, we anticipated sibling interactions would arouse tensions: some deaf siblings objected to their hearing siblings' lack of recognition for the value of their input into the family's decision-making process throughout different periods of their lives. In these situations, these same siblings admitted having felt ambivalent depending on who was involved and their comfort with the topic under discussion. For example, if the discussion centered on an upcoming anniversary party with relatives and inquiries were going around about who would do what for a potluck, if deaf siblings had no knowledge of the prior discussions about the event, it placed them "on the spot," resulting in anxiety or discomfort. Yet there were instances, although not a rarity, where some have expressed deep gratitude for their hearing siblings' efforts to reduce their isolation, feeling content in their dependence on the hearing sibling.

There were also moments of deaf siblings' limited awareness of the effect their reactions might have on the relationship with their hearing siblings. The intensity of their closeness was tied not only to whether isolation was addressed but also to the capacity of the siblings to see one another as siblings first and to accept the deaf status as a neutral attribute.

To combat their deaf sibling's isolation, some hearing siblings interviewed already had an effective tool: sign. These hearing siblings experienced the inherent shortcomings of oral communication and mutually perceived signing as an enormous advantage, especially when accompanied by deaf cultural values. With a common language and cultural competency, without either believing the disability was the culprit for their communication difficulties, they confirmed as siblings they could just be themselves. Conversing in sign as well as embracing deaf culture was a safety net, reducing isolation in hearing environments, urging the siblings to pursue ongoing contact. Engagement in deep, personal conversations allowed them to be equal participants whose stories revealed common interests and explorations of their differences. Their sibling interactions were abundant, filled with details. The nuances of serious business, sarcasm, humor, anger, gentle or subtle teasing, as well as childhood laughter and tears, revealed clear turn-taking, using visual, not auditory cues: waving to get each other's attention, stomping on the floor or flicking the lights. Spontaneity was an integral part of their everyday chatter, in ASL.

The advantages of sharing a common language and embracing one another's auditory and visual behaviors gave the signing siblings what experts in family dynamics believe is the primary role siblings play in one another's lives: the opportunity to learn and develop social skills from one another throughout childhood.

> Parents of children with disabilities also recognize the value of social interaction and wish to optimize social interaction between their children. If the sibling and the child with a disability do not socialize well with each other, the loss of the benefits of such a relationship will be more detrimental for the child with the disability than for the other child. Because the child with a disability may have limited opportunities to interact with other children, social interaction with siblings often takes on increased importance. Efforts to facilitate this interaction will be important to the child's development [Powell and Gallagher 1993, 140].

Those deaf and hearing siblings who shared a common language, with no language barrier isolating them, were involved in each other's lives. Using sign provided ample opportunities to appreciate or disagree with each other's thoughts and opinions. It also guaranteed access to each other's personalities, quirks, and subtleties without being bogged down in struggles to understand or be understood. The deaf sibling trusted and expected the hearing sibling to sign in their presence, presenting a challenge as non-signers joined the family conversations.

During her interview, Darcy shared her concern about whether a future partner would be willing to learn sign to communicate on his own:

> I've always, kind of, been hesitant to tell people about my deaf brother. I don't know why. I'm not ashamed of him. It's not that. Are they going to be sensitive? Or are they going to laugh in my face or are they going to ... not care? I've always

had this fantasy I'm going to marry someone who knows what it's like and who is going to be able to communicate with my brother easily without my having to facilitate it. When I'm first meeting them, I'm thinking, "How will they react to meeting my brother?" And I guess that's how I know. It's like a litmus test, you know.

Siblings tend to be more fluent bilinguals than their parents, especially if their parents learn ASL as a second language. Darcy is a typical bilingual sibling; she acquired Sign and English simultaneously. Both languages are as natural to her as breathing, easily picked up through exposure and immersion. Growing up in this kind of bilingual home gives siblings an opportunity few deaf and hearing siblings ever have, a chance to be intimate in a language they both embraced and where their relationship could flourish.

Characteristic of bilingual children, Haley probably knew exactly when to use Sign with her deaf brother and when to use spoken English with their hearing parents. The siblings who signed didn't choose it; their parents did. By doing so, they affirmed, like several families we interviewed, that signing is a positive, effective way to communicate. Being bilingual does not guarantee a person will be bicultural, adapting the nuances of a native. For instance, a "sibling culture" could be influenced by what is happening "in the moment," where deaf and hearing siblings bring their insider jokes, quirks, habits, and their years of interactions into the relationship. In contrast, siblings or any adults who choose to have a deaf or hearing partner, spouse or family friend may or may not resemble the broad continuum of closeness of the deaf and hearing siblings we interviewed. Are these relationships skewed because they made the choice? When tensions, conflicts, and rivalries arise, which are inevitable, each tends to revert to their language and their culture to address them. Often the ability to communicate becomes the deciding factor that facilitates the cross-cultural parameters as they arise, such as valuing ASL.

A major advantage of using ASL is its unique feature: 3-dimensions, almost like being drawn into a movie. The use of signing space shows ASL users where things are located, physical descriptions of ideas, places, and things, and how they relate to one another. Auditory languages are linear and rarely establish spatial relationships between ideas. Sometimes we say things in ASL in half the time it takes to say it in a spoken language: a picture *is* worth a thousand words. As a visual-spatial language, the signer nurtures the visual and kinesthetic senses when taking on a character role exhibiting the actions in the movie. In addition, as an attractive communication tool, the 3-D feature of ASL provides the pathway for children to make direct emotional connections with the visual images they see in ASL as they engage in conversations with their deaf siblings and other relatives.

A common language is not a panacea. One deaf sibling, Deidre, chronicled instances when her sister Rae would slide back and forth between speaking and Signing using only partial or incorrect signs. As her hearing sibling's main sign coach, Deidre instinctively fed her sister vocabulary to fill in the gaps. This led Rae to realize how frequently Deidre was being left out. To compensate for the isolation she caused, Rae pretended to be deaf, signing only to hearing non-signers, when the two sisters hung out together in public. Deidre believed this behavior *"showed me a lot that she cared about me."* The language was the key, in spite of the absence of deaf cultural aspects, since the environment was predominantly hearing. Rae's "playing deaf" showed that she not only empathized with Deidre's isolation but Rae was able to test out the responses of hearing people in their environment. Each of these encounters is part of Rae's awakening and enculturation to maneuvering the circumstances her sister experiences on a daily basis. Using ASL, Deidre is able to instill the deaf values that are critical to the interaction between the sisters. Deidre's ASL conversations modeled them: open and direct discourse, priority in identifying personal connections with mutual acquaintances, or detailed elaboration about people's lives and daily occurrences.

Other signing sibling pairs had different approaches to some of the nuances that influenced their "common language." Kevin spoke of his preference for ASL but was willing to settle for Signed English; his sister Darcy's ASL and exposure to deaf culture was limited. What mattered more to him was his need to keep himself entertained, by chatting with her, rather than be trapped by the isolation. He said he had been willing to coach her in ASL and even offered himself to serve as an intermediary between his ASL friends and her whenever needed, should any potential cultural clashes occur. One sibling pair who openly discussed strategies to combat the isolation was adamant their use of ASL and adopting some of the cultural behaviors naturally occurring in the DEAF-WORLD was instrumental to their bond. However, realistically they admitted the completeness of the isolation of the deaf sibling went way beyond amelioration by their shared common language and culture.

As witnesses, like bilingual children of immigrants, some hearing siblings felt torn: if they spent time with hearing relatives, they became part of the problem, complicit in isolating their deaf sister or brother. Hearing siblings' anxiety added unnecessary strain to fragile sibling relations, especially at family gatherings. Rae elaborated, *"Sometimes my parents didn't know how to communicate well enough to discipline her. Instead of scrambling to find the Signs, they just let it go. It was like she was an alien. But to me, she wasn't an alien. She was just my sister."* Hearing siblings like Rae were baffled by their parents' ineptness at communicating with their deaf sibling, especially creating tension when deaf siblings received preferential treatment. For second language learners like

Rae's parents, "Learning ASL is the hardest thing for parents will ever do in life" (Solomon 2012, 106), but as a child, Rae acquired Sign from interacting with her sister, unlike the formal aspect of studying in an ASL class.

Hearing siblings' internal struggles—whether to align with hearing relatives or be with deaf siblings—did have positive effects. Aligning themselves with the deaf family member during stressful times, their action reinforced that they were there for the deaf sibling by means of accepting their share of the experience. Furthermore, hearing siblings were somewhat relieved knowing their deaf sibling was less isolated by their presence. Nevertheless, several hearing siblings remained disturbed by an ongoing dilemma: they didn't want deaf siblings to see them as part of the hearing world that isolated them, but the fact remained that they are hearing, and were left wondering, "Where do I belong?" The dilemma is the ambivalence in having to choose between people they love. The ambivalence is no different for deaf siblings choosing between their "homes": the DEAF-WORLD and their hearing family.

Am I My Sister's Keeper?

Each time deaf and hearing siblings experience isolation together, they are churned by the intensity of their reactions: Am I the *only* one who has to do something? Since the emotion is unspoken and rarely addressed, sibling bonds are challenged by the ups and downs of family dramas with years of trial and error, testing the very formation of their alliances. Deaf people live with a unique challenge: lasting ambiguity. Each time isolation rears its ugly head, they wonder whether hearing siblings will come through. Deaf siblings' stories revealed survival tactics from ambiguities and anxieties accompanying relentless encounters with isolation. Yet through years of hit-or-miss experiences, deaf siblings uncovered a host of tools they and their hearing siblings used to secure bonds with one another.

Hearing siblings who witnessed their deaf siblings' isolation could not betray their sister or brother. In 1967, in the midst of the Vietnam War, Martin Luther King, Jr. said, "There comes a time when silence is betrayal" (Strol 2011). Like those who witness bullying, they instinctively knew: bystanders who witness and do nothing are as guilty as the perpetrator, the bully. The majority of hearing siblings believed they were responsible to do something about their deaf siblings' isolation and took action with whatever tools they could muster. Many hearing siblings believed providing access was integral to their role in the family. From the deaf perspective, however, though their hearing sibling's actions were often better than nothing, the actions were neither consistent nor sufficient for the deaf siblings to fully participate, nor did the actions contribute to deaf siblings' developing deeper and closer relationships with relatives or family friends. In addition, the deaf siblings were aware of conflicting feelings: they were never quite sure their sibling *would* provide access.

Some hearing siblings knew if they learned to sign, aligning with deaf siblings to reduce the isolation, other family members wouldn't step up to the plate or share responsibility. Hearing siblings' difficulty centered on this belief: "Once I know the language, I can't go home again; I have a responsibility I can't avoid—responsibility to provide access when I see a deaf person being isolated among hearing people who don't sign." Adding fuel to the fire, some hearing siblings avoided family gatherings, knowing they would feel obligated to provide access by interpreting for many hours. After an onerous lifetime of observing deaf siblings' isolation at family gatherings, several hearing siblings were unable to move beyond their anger; they simply gave up trying to educate relatives and family friends about their deaf siblings' isolation.

Hearing siblings who signed injected instant intimacy into the siblings' relationship, especially at hearing-dominated events where visual cues were not conveyed, like who was interrupting, laughing, or interjecting a comment. At the same time, several deaf siblings became aware of the power hearing siblings held over them. Since hearing siblings were the only ones who heard, saw and understood both languages, they could decide when, where and how much information to give. Only one pair of siblings openly discussed the power imbalance. Nevertheless, the deaf siblings lived with their hearing siblings in control, with the potential to impair childhood and adult relationships. Deidre taught Rae how she was able to get the power back from interference by a hearing interrupter:

> Often when I'm involved in a sign conversation with my sister, a hearing friend or family member would talk to her. Without any warning, I see her turning away, ignoring me and responding to them. I lose patience waiting for us to resume our conversation. This is how I resolve this: I tell her, "Let me finish what I have to say and tell me someone's talking to you, then you can go ahead and listen to them." It's the same idea when people want my attention while I'm signing. I say, "Hold on," and finish signing. My sister said she did not intend to ignore me. She said because she hears them calling to her, she automatically responds and said she could listen to them and me at the same time. But I told her, "No, you need to look at me." My family knows how important eye contact is to me; it shows me they are really listening.

In some families, hearing siblings' providing inconsistent access created a whole range of unresolved emotions and anxieties for the deaf siblings. Several deaf siblings had hearing siblings who were on their side, empathetic allies who understood pain and the disastrous consequences of isolation. These siblings were the only family member who "understood me to the core," like no one else. More importantly, neither was alone; the alliance brought deaf and hearing siblings closer, sharing the common enemy—hearing relatives who just didn't get it. Other deaf siblings knew they couldn't rely on hearing siblings for access at all. The relentless struggles, coupled with lack of reciprocity from hearing siblings, kept these relationships distant, or what Cicirelli and Gold label apathetic, though mutually cordial. For those deaf siblings who used a Band-Aid approach of intermittent access, intimacy with the hearing sibling was a step closer to becoming a possibility. However, deaf siblings lived with ongoing anxiety-producing consequences.

With disbelief, in daily encounters, hearing siblings saw no one else taking action to eliminate their deaf sibling's isolation and thought, "If not me, then who?" Some had to deliberate whether to follow their parents or take their own path. Among those siblings who were raised orally, some stepped up to the plate by mouthing or summarizing what others said. Several siblings' fluency in sign made it possible to provide access their deaf sibling required. Several hearing siblings were appalled that their sign skills surpassed those of their own parents. They were even astonished by their exposure to the DEAF-WORLD. Not only had they learned another language and culture, but socializing with deaf people had enriched their lives. Simultaneously, hearing siblings realized they were in a conundrum: providing access had consequences. Family members and others had no reason to devise their own strategies to have a relationship with the deaf family member. Hearing siblings also discovered they held the power to control and decide what deaf siblings would know about the world around them. Whether to use or abuse the power created an uneven balance of power, which was a deciding factor for how the sibling relationship would evolve: intimate, congenial, loyal, apathetic or hostile (Cicirelli 1995, Gold 1989). Yet if deaf and hearing siblings had meta-conversations about the power imbalance, the discussions could become the gateway for bonding.

Does partaking in shared experiences lead to intimacy? Or does the desire for intimacy lead us to share our love, laughter, joy, grief, fear of the unknown, and so much more? If sibling intimacy entails the baggage inherited from childhood days, when their lives were intertwined with family activities, then what makes it a desirable relationship? We propose intimacy flourishes when there are "equally-powered transactions" (Luterman 1987, 8–9) between siblings accompanied by each holding high regard for "being a sibling." In the deaf and hearing sibling interviews, although each expressed a desire to have a close relationship with their sibling, only a few thought they had attained it. One overarching repeated theme seemed to hover around siblings like a perpetually dark cloud: the deaf sibling's ongoing isolation, and realizing isolation was not a single incident, but a constant occurrence. So profound was the repetitive experience embedded into both deaf and hearing siblings' psyches, it was how they came to be—as a sibling. During the interviews, deaf and hearing siblings discussed how they managed ongoing isolation occurrences—whether alone or as partners—each faced on-the-spot decisions. These decisions most often did not entail a conversation between the siblings about how to combat isolation, pool ideas, resources, or any other tool to get through it. Instead, awareness was the first step toward taking action, followed by the conscious belief that "I am the *only* one who has to do something."

Peeling Off the Deaf Attribution

Since the recurrence of the isolation pervading the deaf family member's life is part of deaf and hearing siblings' experience, what actions do they take to alleviate isolation? And what is the impact of those actions towards the desire for a closer sibling bond? The roles deaf and hearing siblings see themselves taking on in their families are often defined by their relation to one another either as siblings or as deaf and hearing siblings.

The undertakings of communication and isolation were driving forces in our deaf and hearing interviews. Siblings talked at length of strategies they used to alleviate deaf siblings' isolation in settings with non-signers. While describing the strategies, the majority of hearing siblings characterized their roles as follows:

- I was his/her voice.
- I explained to other family members ways to communicate with her/him.
- I kept him/her company.
- I was his/her protector.
- I watched out for him/her.
- I filled her/him in or summarized what others said.
- I interpreted for her/him.

These hearing siblings saw themselves as the sibling of a *deaf* person. Discussions revolved around what they did or did not do for their deaf siblings as a response to communication and relieving isolation—not about who their sibling was as a person who has attributes other than being deaf.

What did deaf siblings say to personalize their roles with respect to their hearing sibling? Instead of describing themselves with clearly defined strategies to combat the communication and isolation issues, several deaf siblings were colonized and victimized by the pathological attribution term—as deaf by the hearing world. Hearing siblings were part of that world, dominating and contributing to deaf siblings' invisibility, making it difficult, if not impossible, for deaf siblings to have a voice or establish their own roles in the family. Since these deaf and hearing siblings were preoccupied with negative attributions, stigmatized by issues surrounding communication and isolation, rarely did they describe their own hobbies, interests, personalities and idiosyncrasies. During the interviews, we pulled teeth trying to get these deaf and hearing siblings past the deaf attribution to share valuable characteristics of sibling relationships other than those related to deaf issues.

The bottom line for us was whether the open-ended interviews, with us as insiders using a conversational format, may have contributed to our impression that both groups of siblings did not get much beyond attribution—seeing one another in specific *deaf* or *hearing* roles first, rather than as their siblings—with a few exceptions. Were they moody, intelligent, good mechanics, generous, skilled in art or ambitious? Knowing these specific traits about one another promotes intimacy, and we were fortunate to have a few who told us about their siblings as well-rounded people—deaf and hearing who are also their siblings.

How do we get past the negative stigma accompanying the attribution of being deaf? In a hearing family, it begins with how family members treat one another. Deaf siblings have been living in deaf shells for eons. Asking them to find who they are as people and as siblings begins at home, the place we humans hope to have unconditional acceptance as a family member where positive attributions define who we are as a *person*. Positive attributions will demolish negative ones, starting with *every* family member, including the deaf siblings.

At the time we conducted our interviews, only a few sibling pairs were content with the relationship they had with one another, that is, falling solidly on the congenial end of Cicirelli and Gold's continuum. With a few exceptions, most expressed desires for a closer bond. Since the siblings seemed to self-describe closeness as it pertained to deaf attribution, we followed their lead, assessing the varying degrees of experience or roles they took on regarding their:

- perspectives on parents' expectations for each sibling

- awareness about the deaf sibling's isolation
- hearing sibling's fluency in ASL

- tools each sibling used to combat communication and isolation issues

- views about each siblings' role in the family with regard to the deaf sibling
- knowledge about ASL, deaf culture, history, and the arts
- hearing sibling's willingness to take action to ameliorate deaf sibling's isolation

Deaf and hearing siblings used different strategies to nurture or obstruct sibling bonds. Our research has clearly identified several sibling pair actions and roles fostering intimacy. Some siblings were more expressive than others, while others with just a few words shared incredible insights. Since intimacy appeared to be connected with deaf attribution, we identified specific actions hearing siblings took on in relationship to their deaf siblings: monitoring, communication facilitating, signing, and interpreting. Our intention is to demonstrate the realities of how deaf and hearing siblings described their relationship to one another at the time they were interviewed. In addition, with great gratitude, we saw what we envisioned as the "sign of things to come" from two sibling pairs: a deep connection with my sibling means, "I accept you for who you are and I expect you will do the same for me."

PART THREE

SIBLING BUDDIES

The Siblings We Could Be

Remember we were sitting on the beach.
Our conversations felt like an eternity but it lasted an hour.
Distractions interjected by the kids and little pooch digging in the sand.
You tuned out sounds of laughter, waves, and millions of conversations.
I traced visual noises of sand grain sprinkles,
    molecule splashes, and bodies wandering around.
As you embraced every breeze, my eyes eagerly ready at every rush.
Not a word was uttered, constant companion was found.
Clammed up, first move was futile yet a possible breakthrough.
Each minute shriveled the gift our parents gave us.
As adults, we were gone long before.
Meta-conversation is the quantum leap,
To be sisters and brothers.

by Marla C. Berkowitz

9

Sibling Monitors

"My sister was part of the popular crowd. She wouldn't bring her friends home. She was embarrassed because I was deaf and not as popular as she was."

—Greg

Deaf and hearing siblings have natural differences in sensitivity to situations around them, along with unique personalities, expectations and interests that easily lead to conflicts, unrelated to isolation of the deaf family member. Each encounter with isolation is unlike any other. For this reason, deaf and hearing siblings get overwhelmed by uncertainty about how to respond—bombarded by their awareness, subsequent feelings and the action they feel forced to take. Although each sibling's response to isolation varied, our interviews revealed common strategies. Action began the moment a hearing sibling moved from being aware of the isolation to monitoring it.

Yet action came with an emotional attachment to the very role siblings play in each other's lives. One hearing sibling, Ginger, explicitly described the dangers of siblings having a dependency relationship.

> As a sibling you can be very enabling and I think it is important to let your sisters and brothers be who they are and have them be your sister or brother first. The balancing act—between being a sibling and taking action—is difficult when one sibling is isolated. The practical response is to do one's best and "deal with it."

Isolation is the "it" that must be addressed. Only one deaf and hearing sibling pair who used ASL had intense conversations by forming a team, strategizing and developing cues to determine when and where the hearing sibling would take steps to monitor the isolation. This deaf sibling, Kay, reminisced about her sister's unwavering commitment: *"At any extracurricular activity, my sister was always there. She always supported me. If I hadn't had my family and my sister's support, I wouldn't have succeeded."* Kay's success was unmistakable. She excelled academically and was a social butterfly at her public high school. The presence of her hearing sister, Bree, as a bystander who did whatever it took, was the equivalent of having someone to count on, and meant that monitoring was an effective tool. These sisters turned the isolation experience into a strategy for support.

In contrast to the deaf-hearing team who benefited from monitoring as an agreed-upon tool, another pair of siblings clashed. One deaf sibling, Terrence, gave an example of how his hearing sibling undermined his independence at a restaurant: "*I would tell her, "It's fine, I can order myself." I point to items on the menu to show the server what I wanted instead of having her speak for me. My sister would be reluctant to go along with what I wanted.*" Although his hearing sibling, Haley, meant well, her monitoring, which had the potential to make a difference, was an ineffective tool, adding strain to the sibling relationship. Over time, trust in monitoring is earned through a gradual process of countless brief interactions, longer dialogues and in-depth conversations. How do these siblings move beyond the potential risks? According to the deaf siblings, every interaction with hearing non-signers is unpredictable. Therefore, effectiveness of monitoring had to be assessed each time for hearing siblings to earn their trust, which depended upon the effectiveness of deaf siblings' communication with non-signers.

Deaf siblings admitted feeling hearing people's interactions with them were not natural and lacked easygoing give and take. Numerous misunderstandings, requiring laborious work from both siblings, created distance. Deaf sibling conversations with hearing people were similar to talking with someone who mumbles, often with innumerable interruptions of "What?" Those kinds of interactions lead either or both to give up, walk away, or at a minimum, restrict themselves to asking short questions with predictable answers. Simultaneously, some deaf siblings we interviewed have often wondered, "Will anybody—most especially my sibling—come along to rescue me so I have a *chance* to get to know my fellow travelers?"

If deaf siblings see hearing siblings as empathetic to their isolation experience, deaf siblings trust them to monitor and come to believe the hearing sibling will be there for them. When communication barriers continue to occur—such as lack of proficiency in sign, lipreading or speech—conversational spontaneity is unlikely. The unease of interaction defeats the effectiveness of using monitoring as a tool to sustain trust in creating or establishing sibling bonds.

To illustrate, there are deaf individuals who have confidence lipreading their siblings while simultaneously have little faith in expressing themselves using speech. When they repeat or rephrase words, or sometimes even resort to writing, others may or may not understand them. The reverse also occurs:

an individual's speech may be understood, but lipreading is an insurmountable obstacle. Since only one-third of spoken language is seen on lips, deaf people with no or limited residual hearing expend energy just trying to decipher lip movements. It becomes insignificant to even ask deaf or hard-of-hearing persons if they lipread. They must, if they are going to get anything from face-to-face conversations with non-signers. Yet guessing plays such a large role they barely have a chance to process what they are seeing, let alone get nuances of tone like sarcasm, humor or boredom. At least one of the perks of being a hearing sibling is that the years of practice deciphering their deaf siblings' speech, develops their lipreading skills to supplement what they hear. In addition, they find these skills useful when they are in noisy environments.

Additional barriers do present themselves if struggles continue to inhibit conversations between deaf and hearing siblings. Time is wasted figuring out what the other is signing or saying. Feelings of torment surface at the lack of easy give and take, and deaf siblings' irritation at hearing siblings' unwillingness to address mutual struggles to communicate grows. These consequences have proven to devastate deaf siblings' sense of security in their rapport. More specifically, the outcome affirmed by the deaf siblings in conversations with hearing siblings are often superficial, predictable, limited and shallow, all of which lead to questionable trust as it applies to using monitoring as a tool. The critical feature is both siblings' desire to feel at ease, confidently expressing themselves fully—their deepest thoughts, dreams, and opinions—without struggling to understand or be understood.

Other deaf siblings, even though they never openly discussed the topic, expressed their contentment with monitoring, the way the hearing sibling "watched out for me." It could mean having a sibling on the lookout for you, just as a parent would for a child. This fictionalized story, "Signing Family," provides insight to how a hearing sibling looks out for the deaf sibling, perhaps no differently from the way an older sibling protecting a younger sibling. Yet underlying this protectiveness are sensitivities surrounding the effectiveness of monitoring the communication among the family members and non-signers.

Signing Family

After the car maneuvered into the parking space, the family stumbled out of the car, exhausted from a whirlwind day of shopping. As Rachel entered the restaurant lobby, she reminded her sister Chloe, "Don't forget to ask the server for a round table." They looked around the room as the hostess said, "Four?"

In the center of each table was a tall vase holding an assortment of daisies, asters and marigolds. As soon as Rachel and Chloe sat down, signing and speaking simultaneously, Rachel handed the flowers to the hostess: "These will block our conversation. They're pretty but they have to go."

While they were waiting for their drinks, Rachel, looking at the menu, finger-spelled, "What's C-A-P-E-R-S?"

Chloe hesitated. "Hmm. They're hard to explain," as her hands drew a picture in the air of a plant stem with tiny green circles hanging from it.

Rachel responded: "Oh, do they taste of vinegar? I've seen them! Is that the name?"

Mr. Hampton turned to his wife and spoke, without signing, "What are you folks gabbing about? You know, it's often hard for me to follow when the three of you are signing so fast."

Mrs. Hampton replied, "Me too! Sometimes I can't always catch what these girls are signing. Anyway, Chloe's thinking of having broiled shrimp and Rachel didn't know what capers were, so Chloe explained."

Chloe tapped Rachel's shoulder, "See, I told you. Dad couldn't understand us and asked Mom what we were talking about. And she A-D-M-I-T she get lost E-A-V-E-S-D-R-O-P us. Ha ha!"

Rachel smiled. "Sign this for admit and eavesdrop."

"Hi, my name is Barbara. I'm your server today. What can I get for you?" Her head turned to Chloe, whose hands were flying in the air.

Chloe signed "WHICH SOUP, SALAD WHICH? Barbara ran off her list of soup options, but Chloe lagged behind, juggling the signs or fingerspelling words while speaking Rachel's preferred choice.

Orders were still going around until Chloe's turn came. She took a deep breath, Signing and speaking simultaneously, "I'd like the shrimp salad with ranch dressing on the side." She fingerspelled S-H-R-I-M-P.

"Dammit, Rachel, I knew that sign!"

Rachel signed rapidly, "Come on, don't be so hard on yourself. Mom would have forgotten the sign too!"

Chloe replied: "Right on! Even though Mom took Sign classes! What's funny, she tried teaching Grandma and Grandpa, and I think Aunt Carol and Uncle John too. Sometimes they were so dense, they couldn't figure out what you were saying."

Rachel gasped, "Really? I didn't know!"

Chloe interrupted, "But it was simple, like the sign for drinking from a glass ... like you wanted something to drink. It was bizarre that they couldn't get it!"

As they waited for their food to arrive, Mr. and Mrs. Hampton were deep in conversation. Chloe's eyes were concentrated on them. Rachel curiously looked around the restaurant, examining the chatting families. Chloe caught herself and explained to Rachel, "They're figuring out what to do with grandma's house, probably meaning they'll sell it."

A moment later, Rachel caught the server's eye, waving her over. Carefully she enunciated, "Where's the bathroom?"

"What?" Barbara replied.

Chloe looked up and turned to Rachel, "What'd you want?"

"The bathroom."

Chloe said, "She'd like to know where the ladies' room is.... Ok. Thank you so much."

As Barbara left, Chloe pointed at the restroom sign way up front, near the cashier. When Rachel came back, she saw Chloe chuckling.

Rachel's head started to turn around but Chloe's hand caught her eye, "Stop! Don't look behind you!" and continued Signing.

The sisters burst out laughing. Mr. Hampton looked over at them and glared. Mrs. Hampton giggled and whispered in his ear, "This time I got it. They're just eavesdropping on the people behind Chloe about some stuff going on at a hangout downtown."

Families who sign may not be common, but in this family both Rachel and her family members have accepted sign as the norm. This family's experience in a public place is typical of families whose parents have chosen to sign, when the hearing sibling takes on the monitoring role instead of the parents. Research shows young children acquire languages more readily than adults who are second language learners.[1]

In this brief segment, Chloe, the hearing sibling, was attuned and alert to their parents and other diners' conversations by summarizing in Sign what she overheard. Her sister Rachel was fully aware of the conversations occurring, yet she was stumped by the context: the *who, when where* and/or *why*. In addition, as soon as Chloe heard Rachel's voice, she took action to ensure Rachel was accessible to the hearing server, Barbara. The responsibility for monitoring, falling on Chloe, appears to be one-sided. However, the intimate interaction between sisters is ripe for trust-building: Rachel gains access to learning new information each time Chloe Signs the surrounding comments from external conversations. Trust is earned when two sisters participate in the shared happening, instead of one sister living the experience alone in her sister's presence. By taking action, beginning with monitoring, the sisters guarantee opportunities for bonding.

Chloe notices Rachel uses her as a default communicator, yet she worries a lot. Each time they are together, Chloe wonders whether she is Signing correctly. However, she is grateful Rachel is willing to continue to feed her correct vocabulary. For Rachel, all that mattered was to communicate effectively with non-signers; thus, she was willing to overlook Chloe's mediocre Signing skills. On the other hand, Rachel's dependency on Chloe has the potential to diminish Rachel's confidence in her communication with hearing people. These sisters may be at a crossroads, yearning to be close, yet instances of potential isolation continue to challenge them daily. Both sisters want Rachel to be independent in the presence of hearing people. The reality is they have not yet found the tools to achieve a mutual goal.

Despite the issues, Chloe and Rachel share a common language and they have communicated effectively since they were children. As adults, they have baggage that looks like a deaf issue, because it manifests itself around Chloe's signing for Rachel. However, in the general scheme of sibling issues, Chloe's protective behavior towards Rachel could be just one sibling trying to help another avoid pain or embarrassment. Is it any different from one sibling advising or assisting another on how to dress, put on make-up or shoot a basket? These two siblings have a close and loving relationship. The commitment by the hearing sibling to sign is a tool that nourishes the opportunities life presents. Knowing they might have challenges in communicating with non-signers in the restaurant, they used monitoring as the relief to manage potential isolation. Monitoring to deaf siblings is personal: like having someone sitting on your shoulder.

Other deaf siblings had varied comments based on their experiences with siblings' monitoring:

> JOY: My sister wouldn't let me talk to my friend. My sister thought it was a stranger on the street.
> BROOKE: I don't know if they do it or not. Sometimes, I wish I knew.
> JARON: My sister should be watching out for me. She knows it is difficult for me to participate in family conversations.

The common thread of their responses indicates anxiety accompanying potential misunderstood intentions. None of these deaf siblings considered the hearing siblings' role as a monitor, but just as something a sibling does or should do.

Bubble Talk

Family gatherings epitomize deaf family members' isolation—alone in a room filled with hearing, non-signing relatives. One sibling pair we met had a powerful tool to combat the division at family gatherings. It's almost a weapon: *"She knows I'm watching out for her." Knowing* meant Kay was now part of the conversation with both siblings processing the monitoring.

> Yes, my sister is very aware and she feels it and we both feel it and at the end of the day we always talk about it. So we're like this little bond, a little bubble when we go to family things. We're watching out for each other ... she knows I'm watching out for her. She knows how I feel ... she knows how mad I am.
>
> We have that open communication. So I know she ... doesn't want me to "have to" interpret. Sometimes we get into a debate about it ... so I am comfortable leaving her and I'm comfortable knowing that if she really needs me, she'll call me, because she does.

The tool starts out in Bree's possession; she's watching. What happens next is a team effort uniting the siblings against the pain of divided family gatherings.

They form their own little "world" and process together what had happened, explore how they feel, and strategize how to handle the inevitable next time.

It seems so simple, but these were the only siblings who said they had worked together to address painful family gatherings. Bree described what she did, using the word *watch,* but she did far more. A more descriptive term for her behavior is *monitor:* "to watch, keep track of, or check usually for a special purpose."[2]

The hearing sibling's monitoring used implicit knowledge, not conscious but rumbling around in her head. Bree's antennas went up in a crowd of hearing relatives, none of whom knew much about deaf people or ASL. Always alert, eyeballing her sister's interactions, she was like an inspector, checking for communication breakdowns. Was Kay not catching a hard-to-lipread word on Grandma's lips? Or was Uncle Matt not deciphering her sister's deaf speech? For sure, her deaf sister didn't know about the loud crash in the kitchen when, while engrossed in a conversation, Aunt Gabriella suddenly disappeared. Bree was always there for Kay, ready to support her, be her ally and minimize her isolation. The attributes of monitoring—a quick cue, a puzzled look or a sign—and Bree, on guard, would drop whatever she was doing. Even while the two sisters were chatting in sign, the hearing sibling was eavesdropping on other conversations, in case a juicy piece of gossip appeared, to share later. She might overhear someone making fun of her deaf sister. The difference between Bree and the other hearing siblings we interviewed was she would later tell her deaf sister about it.

Bree was not the only sibling who monitored. Most of the hearing siblings described behavior fitting the monitoring definition; none used the word. They also reported paying attention to what deaf siblings were doing, noticing whether they were off in a corner, staring out the window, reading a book or watching television. They were keenly aware when the deaf sibling missed an aunt's outrageous story that resulted in fits of laughter throughout the group, and might have tried to retell the story to their deaf sibling. Visible evidence of hearing siblings' monitoring only occurred when they took action.

In the hands of sisters and brothers, monitoring one another is used for protection. Val said she ordered a friend out of her house when he made fun of her deaf brother's voice. Others overheard relatives or neighbors mock their deaf sibling and went to adults for support. Although it was not always forthcoming, it took courage to confront the situation. A few spoke about friends trying to blame deaf siblings for pranks but hearing siblings knew the truth and defended their deaf sibling.

What drives monitoring is the emotional attachment to the deaf sibling. Sibling monitoring is proactive, a result of the personal investment individuals have in their siblings and their insights, precisely because they are family. Siblings have an intimate bond. Monitoring comes from a belief that the deaf sibling is entitled to develop relationships with relatives; proactively they both monitor to assist in that goal. During monitoring, many thoughts race through hearing siblings' minds. If they spot a misunderstanding, confusion, cultural gap or a cue from their deaf sibling, as siblings they have choices: "Do I offer assistance? Give up what I'm doing? Or do nothing?" Regardless of the decision, while they are monitoring, they are rarely relaxed. The "special purposes" always accompany emotionally invested hearing siblings at family gatherings. Their deaf sibling's relentless isolation symbolizes the oppression: that's what the anger is about when Kay said, *"She knows how mad I am."*

In contrast, other siblings we interviewed saw deaf siblings' stagnant relationships with relatives who simply did not know how to interact with a deaf person. Looking out for their deaf sister or brother was a way hearing siblings handled the helpless and painful feelings about their own privileged relationships with extended family members. One hearing sibling, Shari, confessed monitoring for reasons she knew were no longer applicable: *"My role in the family as a child was to watch out for my deaf brother and be his voice."* She admitted that now, as an adult, she was overprotective, always waiting for the next shoe to drop, believing the world was not a deaf-friendly place. Like several other siblings who had been given the caretaker or rescuer role as children, she was struggling to change lifetime habits. Nevertheless, for the most part, hearing siblings believed monitoring, coupled with supportive actions, engendered trust and fostered close ties with their deaf sibling. The kind of monitoring described earlier, the safe bubble of a deaf and hearing sibling partnership, provides a model safety net where both share the vicissitudes and realities living in a sound-dominated world.

However, monitoring is not without its drawbacks. The very act of monitoring—keeping track for a special purpose—is a stressful undertaking, requiring psychic energy devoted to continual decision-making about deaf siblings' well-being. Even if deaf siblings are aware of the stress, sometimes seen as a burden, monitoring comes from deep affection marking a desire for closeness in the relationship. It also has consequences, especially if the monitor decides to act without a signal from the deaf sibling. One easily overlooked drawback is the potential for the deaf and hearing non-signing participants to believe there is no incentive to formulate their own strategies.

Other hearing siblings acknowledged, with their minds elsewhere and eyes on their deaf sibling, that they gave up opportunities for their own quality time with relatives who do not Sign. Over time, unless deaf and hearing siblings found a satisfactory balance, where resentment might trump monitoring and its subsequent actions, the emotional consequences of remaining silent might not be a price they'd be willing to pay. After observing her deaf sibling's isolation at innumerable family gatherings, one sibling, Noelle, admitted if she learned ASL, it would have consequences she didn't relish: *"Am I then going to have to be the interpreter everywhere we go? So that it becomes my responsibility to make sure my brother knows what's going on and that takes away from me."* Another professional interpreter we interviewed recognized, from monitoring, how few relatives interacted with a deaf sibling without her involvement, leaving her angry at their unwillingness to make any effort to sign or find ways to interact on their own. The common thread of most monitoring efforts is the hearing siblings' response to feeling responsible for ameliorating deaf siblings' isolation. They are outnumbered by the vast majority of family members who do not recognize the existence of the isolation, the monitoring efforts and the subsequent actions taken by the hearing siblings. It's as if these things had no connection to them, rarely considered on their radar screen as shared responsibilities among all family members.

A final drawback associated with monitoring was the ongoing internal struggle to decide whether or when to educate people about ways to interact with the deaf sibling. What seemed so natural to hearing siblings didn't come automatically to people who didn't grow up with a deaf brother or sister. Maintaining vigilance, keeping an eye on the deaf sibling while debating whether or not to intervene, remained a constant challenge at restaurants, extended family gatherings, and family vacations, particularly in places where people might not be aware that their siblings were deaf.

The bottom line, however, is whether monitoring is an effective tool. From the hearing sibling's perspective, monitoring works. It leads deaf siblings to more gratifying interactions, rather than communication breakdowns. Monitoring combats deaf siblings' isolation and, perhaps, most importantly, cultivates harmony. "It is not the presence of conflict in a family that determines its health but rather how the conflicts are resolved" (Luterman 1987, 59). The presence of conflict in families with deaf and hearing siblings tend to revolve around communication breakdowns and using the *deaf card* as an excuse. Resolving conflicts entails having numerous ongoing conversations. How can deaf and hearing siblings resolve their conflicts when frequently they are preoccupied with trying to grasp garbled words or phrases the other is saying or signing, let alone get the ideas, opinions or thoughts expressed? One way to assess whether monitoring achieves trust is to determine, if possible, to what extent the deaf sibling accepts the hearing sibling's judgment and subsequent decision to take action, or resents their hearing sibling not providing support.

10

Sibling Facilitators

"The most vivid memory of growing up with my brother is his love for the beat of loud music. When he was away at school, he'd send me songs, I'd transcribe the lyrics and then he'd sign them to his deaf friends."

—Tara

During the interviews, not all deaf and hearing siblings shared their insiders' bubble talk with us, but we know it exists in different ways. Most siblings just groped for ways to keep the deaf sibling in the loop of chaotic family chatter. In their own ways, both deaf and hearing siblings tried to facilitate the flow of the conversations by filling in missing pieces as best they could.

More often than not, non-signing hearing siblings took over the reins, facilitating the communication using whatever tools they could think of on the spot. The goal was to avoid the hardships caused by potential misunderstandings. Deaf siblings are no strangers to using facilitators at work or in community settings. But hearing siblings performed a different function. Each time hearing siblings, who did not sign, saw their deaf sibling miss a remark or a tidbit, many jumped in without a second thought, to fill them in, especially at home or at family gatherings. In the business world, facilitators' roles are clearly defined and have a purpose: to assist people in strengthening their capacities. Often facilitators support people during individual and group processes, to ensure effective communication and to get people to reflect on what they experienced. Siblings had their own way of describing strategies, often depending on the circumstances, whether it was during mealtimes, a family reunion, or any place when the sibling was the only deaf person present.

Perhaps Aunt Nicole was laughing or gramps looked like he was about to get mad. A quick glance at the deaf sibling's face led some hearing siblings to summarize what was missed. Although the deaf siblings confided that an interpreted summary was nothing like getting it firsthand, some tolerated it because something was better than nothing, which would have escalated their isolation. Keenly aware of the difficulties deaf siblings experienced at extended family gatherings, several hearing siblings took it upon themselves unilaterally to accompany their deaf sibling, explaining who various relatives were and giving information about individuals' lives. These strategies also involved attempts to educate relatives, friends, and sometimes even parents, on how to approach and speak to deaf siblings: *"Face my brother; talk naturally instead of shouting; make clear lip movements without exaggerating; and don't talk with a cigarette or gum in your mouth."* However, despite their best efforts, hearing siblings eventually realized as adults that gestures, home signs,[1] finger-spelling, throwing in a missed word here or there, writing notes back and forth, and/or using Cued Speech, wouldn't make up for a lifetime of deaf siblings' limited relationships with these strangers.

In contrast, the goal of professional facilitators is to inspire people and engage them in thoughtful discussions leading to action. Facilitators take their work seriously by providing a safe place for individuals to make eye contact with one another, inviting smooth reciprocity among participants. Monitoring body language, facilitators ensure approachability, conveying their tone as calm, yet energetic. However, non-signing hearing siblings seldom had a specific agenda. According to the deaf siblings, hearing siblings did know to face them, assuring eye contact, but body language and overall affect, or tone, was absent. Deaf siblings also facilitated communication between their deaf friends and their hearing siblings. Without hesitation, they too jumped in, elaborating or summarizing what their deaf friends were saying, so their hearing siblings would be part of their loop.

Our interviews provide evidence of siblings who took on the responsibility of ensuring effective communication. Some told how they challenged their parents' behavior by acting on their own, and others described how they copied their parents' model, to provide access for their deaf sibling. The act of monitoring and facilitating access for their deaf sisters and brothers may be perceived as too much to expect from a child, especially when the adults can barely deal with the obligation themselves. However, the fact remains that many took it upon themselves and took it for granted, as part of their growing up as a sibling. Perhaps these actions stemmed from conflicting messages from their parents: You are a kid but you are to watch out for your sibling. We believe this is simply another long list of teaching moments parents typically confront with their children: don't hurt your sibling, resolve your own fights, share with or take care of your sibling. Often siblings are not even aware of the responsibilities they undertook until they reach adulthood. Marla's brother,

Joseph, admits his difficult attempts to include her: "*I typically played the role of a poor interpreter—filtering conversations rather than communicating word for word. Back then I felt like I was doing right, yet reflecting back on that—it was probably frustrating for you.*" Their sister Julie agrees:

> At family gatherings, everyone basically just chats away. I see my sister's eyes darting back & forth trying to take all the words, innuendos & information in. It is disturbing to me that she misses content. I always feel responsible to explain & interpret.... I do have memories of being embarrassed when people stared at my need to translate. But I also feel badly because my explanation is in my own words & not the objective version of a true interpreter....

Marla's siblings aren't off base, which probably led to the distancing between her and her hearing siblings:

> We simply didn't have the natural give-and-take I observed in my hearing siblings' spoken interactions. I felt their hesitation or their unwillingness to even broach certain subjects, because the three of us knew I would interrupt with "What?" a thousand times, to catch a confusing word or phrase on their ever-moving lips. I suspect they were probably overwhelmed with the effort required to get their ideas across to me, while I was dying for more, craving connections for them to see me as a valuable presence in their lives. I felt equally exasperated and used similar strategies. Eventually, I've let it go and don't even bother these days.

As children, Marla and her siblings like others in non-signing families didn't have the tools to clearly define and effectively be or use a facilitator. When siblings are engaged in facilitation, dialogue is encouraged by setting agreements, using visual aids and applying different techniques for listening skills. None of these were considered; perhaps no one in the family knew how to initiate a conversation about the issue.

Despite their well-meaning attempts, non-signing hearing siblings were totally oblivious to how their taboo phrases of "Never mind," "It's not important," or "I'll tell you later," alienated their deaf siblings. How is it possible for deaf siblings to look forward to dinnertime as family time if they internalize these taboo phrases and continue to be in the presence of family, but not present? Jaron reminisced:

> There were rules when we could leave—after everyone has finished eating. When I was about 14 or 15 years old, I rebelled. I said, "What for? I don't understand what you're saying." My parents punished me by sending me to my room. I didn't care because my room had a captioned TV and reading my book was better than sitting there. My siblings complained, "It wasn't fair!"

Perhaps Jaron was content with the end result—getting out of there—since rarely was anyone willing to *continually* facilitate his involvement. More than the issue of who would be doing it, every time this happens, tensions between the siblings have the potential to explode. The punishment of the rebel avoids confronting the real issue: the family's inability to look into its communication patterns. Deaf family members are entitled to be part of family conversations, not isolated in their rooms or at the table. The inevitable result is siblings' resentment towards one another escalating over time, possibly years.

In contrast to the above scenario where no effort at facilitation was made, from the deaf sibling's perspective, hearing siblings often use summaries as a response to deaf siblings' requests. Well-meaning attempts had mixed results:

"What are all of you talking about?" Xena asked her brother, who was sitting next to her. "You all seem excited about some place you're going, right? Is it an important occasion?"

"No, not really," he turned to face her. "I'm just filling them in about our plans for this summer. Marlene and I are thinking about Colorado."

The deaf siblings we met chronicled numerous instances like this one. After Xena had missed huge segments leading to the main topic of a discussion, the four-second summary—the abbreviated version—did no justice to information-sharing as part of giving and taking. The hearing sibling's abbreviated version was a monologue rather than a dynamic progression that occurs in a dialogue. Attempts at facilitation omitted all the details, nuances and enthusiasm, leaving deaf siblings, once again invisible, the last ones to know—exacerbating their isolation. It was the equivalent of a slap in the face. Why bother to ask? It made more sense to retreat to other activities: clean up the kitchen or play with cousins and appear busy, rather than stick around only to get vapid summaries. As trivial it may be, facilitation as a tool had dashed deaf siblings' hopes for participation so many times, it lost its appeal. Once again, deaf siblings were betrayed by its failure.

For facilitation to be successful, the tasks that accompany ease of communication include setting specific goals among parties with a time frame. Since deaf and hearing siblings had never had a conversation about goals with each other, hearing siblings' attempts to facilitate inclusion happened spontaneously and unpredictably, in the moment. If these siblings, deaf and hearing, took the time to evaluate the process, they might have had an eye on the fairness of turn-taking in discussion, set up terms of respect in the communication process, encouraged brainstorming ideas and issues, and then summarized what was discussed to stay focused as participants. Instead, facilitation left deaf siblings stuck in reaction mode, trying to respond to what the hearing sibling did, instead of both siblings being part of the solution in the first place.

At best, not only did deaf siblings respond with resilience, they adapted by keeping themselves occupied, bringing a deaf friend, or sometimes refusing even to attend events, avoiding family altogether. Sometimes hearing siblings kept deaf siblings company for a while at a family gathering, offering temporary relief. If hearing siblings gave other family members advice on how to interact with them, it often backfired because the deaf sibling was uncomfortable with the explanations, since they were never asked for their thoughts on the subject. Both siblings noticed how some family members seemed awkward discussing issues related to being deaf. The taboo stemming from the stigma attached to people with disabilities slams the door against resolving the inherent communication challenges.

In spite of mediocre attempts at inclusion by hearing siblings, deaf siblings remain steadfast in their beliefs: being surrounded by family members is all that matters. This fictionalized story, "The Comfort of Status Quo," illustrates the anticipation that goes on before, during and after a family gathering.

THE COMFORT OF STATUS QUO

Micki and her best friend Karen had been down this road before. They sat in their usual places, opposite one another on the bus, chatting and laughing, oblivious to the other passengers. Micki knew what was coming next: the usual after-church Sunday family gathering. She was deep in thought. These Sunday gatherings had become a family tradition and it was unthinkable not to be there. But, when she got there, it was never right.

Suspending her reverie, Micki felt a breeze on her face. Karen's hand was waving, "Earth to Micki!" The two burst out laughing, creating a scene as fellow passengers' heads turned in their direction.

"My gosh, they're staring at us. Anyway, you know how much I dread going through this again," Micki signed with one hand, real low and fast.

"But you have Enid; she is really cool," Karen tried to reassure her. "I am looking forward to seeing her again."

"Yeah, I love my sister, but you know she doesn't sign at all," Micki replied, rolling her eyes. "What's more, I don't expect it to happen any time soon."

Micki looked at her watch, realizing it was getting near the time church services would be ending. "Thank goodness I don't join them at church anymore. I must tell you of my church escapades!"

Karen's eyes widened. "How did you do it? I bet you got caught, right?"

"Yup, it was worth it. They gave up. They didn't know what to do with a deaf kid like me. You know my parents are from the Caribbean and they go to church all the time, like every Sunday, never missing. My oldest sister, Enid, told me that our parents moved to the States to have better opportunities for us kids. So for them, church on Sunday was a little piece of the Caribbean in the U.S."

"Yeah, when we were kids there was no such thing as an interpreter at religious services, like there are today. I have vivid memories of my family belonging to a deaf temple watching a hearing rabbi who had mediocre Signing skills and my parents, siblings and I would just watch him Sign everything from the prayer book. He just graduated from rabbinical school and a deaf member would teach him Sign. Now, we have deaf rabbis!"

"Well, as a kid, even I had more hearing than I have now but there was no way I was gonna follow any of it. I remember when I was younger, I always brought a book with me to read. Always. I was so bored! You know the big hymn book churches have? Anyway, it was big enough to hide a comic book. Sometimes I'd even bring a novel. The people sitting behind me would see me but I didn't care. I had to do something, otherwise I'd go insane. Ya know, lipreading church services were impossible. Sometimes I would go upstairs."

"What was upstairs?"

"The room upstairs was mostly empty. If the main sanctuary was full, people could sit up there. Sometimes I would disappear and go up to that area."

"Did your family know where you went?"

Micki smirked, "No, I think not."

"I guess you had so many sisters and brothers, your parents didn't even notice you were missing."

"Probably. Or they were too busy praying!" Micki chuckled.

Karen nodded with laughter. "You remind me of the many hours I spent in the bathroom with another deaf friend when my parents made me go to synagogue with them! Anyway, go on with your story!"

"OK, be patient. I'm getting there! Many times, one of the Sunday school teachers who knew me would notice I was missing. She made it her business to find me! I would curse under my breath when she forced me to go downstairs where I'd sulk in my seat for the rest of the service. Or, like you, sometimes I would stay in the bathroom for a long time."

Micki glanced outside, as the bus lurched along. "Hey, we need to get off at the next corner. Pull the cord!" Micki signed.

As soon as they entered the house, Micki noticed her brother Drew in the living room, with a cigarette dangling. "What's up, sis?" Drew asked.

"Anything new? And who's your friend?" Just as Micki was about to answer, Enid walked by carrying a tray of cheese and crackers. Angrily she turned to Drew, "Take that cigarette out of your mouth while you're talking. You know Micki is hard of hearing and can't see your lips."

Enid fumed at Micki, "Will he ever learn? How many times do I have to tell him?"

Turning towards Drew, Enid added, "Don't forget to enunciate clearly," as she continued towards the dining room.

"Hey Karen, did you catch what Enid said? She spoke so quickly but it seemed she was complaining about Drew."

"No, but look ... his ciggie's gone! I bet your sister ordered him to do it."

Micki sighed: "Of course, she always watches over me. But the thing is, she still thinks I'm hard of hearing, not deaf! Just because I speak doesn't mean I hear conversations. Sometimes I know someone's talking, but don't catch what they're saying. I've had it with reminding her. And the rest of the family—we've seen this before. None of them sign. Why bother chasing these conversations when they're so superficial? It's always that way. Nothing changes. We'll stay for an hour or so, okay?"

"Yeah, no problem. You really can see this is a hearing house where there's no open space for everyone to see one another. And what's more, the TVs are turned on, but I don't see any captions."

"Yup, and they know, every Sunday, I'm here. You'd think they'd at least do that since I wanna watch the game a bit too."

Suddenly, Enid rushed over to Micki, "You'd never believe this! Mom just told me Jackie decided to go back to Weight Watchers!" and zoomed off to get the phone.

Micki chuckled and signed to Karen, "Our sister Jackie wants to lose weight so now she's back at Weight Watchers."

Karen gasped, "Oy vey! It's her third time, right? Anyway, you're lucky to have Enid. I see she keeps you in the loop. Not like my sister. We're so different. She keeps everything to herself."

Micki nodded. "You're so right about Enid, but I do wish we didn't have to go through her. I've been telling her, since we were kids, so she knows how left out I feel at these weekly gatherings of relatives and friends. Yet, I've missed out on all of Dad's adventures. Today, I still only get a piece of this or that—from Enid, which is better than nothing, but I wish she'd ..."

Karen interrupted, "Of course, Enid could learn ASL! I remember last year she was excited when she showed us her ASL books."

"Yeah, unfortunately, she never practiced. Her excuse was she's busy with taking care of her children, her job at the office and her church thing. So, she complains about finding the time to take ASL classes. And ... who will practice with her since I live an hour away?"

Karen looked puzzled. "But I remember she came to your party two weeks ago. She looked astonished at everyone using ASL, assuming we all were deaf, only to find out some were hearing friends of yours. It seemed to me she was embarrassed she hadn't learned ASL yet."

"Yeah, I really wish she would make it a priority."

The sibling Enid represents was the only hearing interviewee who unpretentiously believed that her excuses weren't convincing, when she said: "*I know ASL is her language and she needs me to learn it. It is a huge part of her culture and I admire it enormously. But ... I am so ashamed. I should be able to talk to her in whatever way she would like.*"

Two sisters, deaf and hearing, obviously love one another and want to strengthen their relationship. A closer look at childhood baggage might give some insights into the roles that have developed in this family and the boundary lines they have become accustomed to using. The oldest sister Enid, Micki's confidante, was the family intermediary, smoothing the way for the other hearing siblings and parents to interact with her deaf sister. Based on our interviews, since the hearing sibling became the intermediary out of necessity, there were mixed responses regarding deaf and hearing siblings' feelings toward its role. On the other hand, we have no way of knowing whether extended family members appreciate the intermediary.

Who wants to be stuck in the middle of family drama? Adding to the complexity is Enid's struggle to take on learning ASL as a priority, making it harder for Enid to ameliorate the isolation Micki experiences in their large family. Wearing the educator's hat to constantly remind family members has become second-nature to Enid. However, the interference jeopardizes exactly what Micki craves: a *direct* relationship with family members. It is essential to see the correlation of events leading Enid to take on other roles in the family. Because she had been summarizing conversations surrounding them, she naturally became the facilitator and advocate for Micki. Help is second nature to her; she does it with her own family and her church. Micki gradually expected more from Enid, especially since others show so little effort. When Enid scolds their brother Drew about speaking with a cigarette in his mouth, Micki has further assurance of Enid's support. But the support for Micki gets diminished each time Enid's actions conflict with Micki's access. For example, using words like *hard of hearing* instead of *deaf*, or talking too fast, making lipreading difficult, all create tensions. Actions do hurt. Enid has not acquired the knowledge or awareness of Micki's pain every time she does it, despite many reminders potentially obstructing the sisters' desire to move their relationship forward.

Since Enid has not learned ASL and other family members don't recognize Micki's need for communication access, whose responsibility is it? Micki normally interacts with her relatives one-on-one, using speech, but the responsibility for communication through lipreading what others are saying is on her shoulders. Her frustration level is at its breaking point. In spite of these feelings, she loves seeing her family and goes every week, even if interactions consist of bland, superficial greetings. What does Micki do with her failed efforts, and how is she expecting to cope when her efforts don't look promising? What Micki does is compromise. She brings a deaf friend, Karen, whose presence may make a dent in the pain. Her friend gives her emotional support in their shared language, diminishing the isolation. Micki's anger at being left out is just beneath the surface. When she says, *"It's always that way. Nothing changes,"* she is resigned, but she admits being good at masking her anger and the pain, making light of both just to survive being with her family. What are the responses of family members when they see her friend? Is she just another body at the gathering, easily blending in with the others?

Only Enid seems to understand why Karen is there. She knows Karen gives Micki the human connection necessary to have healthy perspectives in social settings. Enid is fully aware Micki does not interact with family and friends gathered every Sunday in the same way she had seen when Micki is in her signing crowd. They both know Micki's compromise only perpetuates the cycle of isolation and minimal connections with her siblings and other relatives. Until something changes, Micki and Enid's relationship will remain status quo.

Non-signers like Enid are complex human beings, holding seemingly opposing views at the same time: cognitive dissonance. Even though Enid was Micki's best defender, advocating for Micki's inclusion in family discussions, the fact remained she was a hearing sibling who didn't value ASL enough to make the leap to learn it. On Cicirelli and Gold's continuum of closeness, the sisters were somewhere between loyal and apathetic, though both yearned for more intimacy. Marla's sister Julie had similar advice:

> [A]nyone interacting with a deaf person ... is not to demand that the language be your own. The best communication is a mutual language ... asking the deaf person how he/she feels the communication will be most successful.... But my guess is that learning sign is likely the best tool.... I would advise that the child be taught to speak, since the ability to communicate with the hearing world is an invaluable tool in life.... A deaf child should be able to express thoughts freely in his/her own language. The hearing family members should "speak" that very same language too.

Enid and Julie, like other non-signing siblings, clearly articulated what was missing. However, for whatever reasons, *as adults* they chose not to take the route necessary to have a shared language both needed—ASL—and neither was able to get beyond their parents' model.

Perhaps learning ASL as an adult is like carrying a heavy jug of water to survive the desert. Several deaf siblings kept returning to family gatherings, believing above all that "family is important." On Cicirelli and Gold's continuum, they wavered back and forth between Loyal and Apathetic, sometimes believing that blood is thicker than water, but other times dismissing the idea and turning to deaf peers. Missing the give-and-take in their families and failing to get much from non-signing siblings, they found it elsewhere: in the DEAF-WORLD.

11

Signing Siblings

"My deaf brother and I burst out laughing when I told the server,
'Look mister, my brother is visually impaired and I'm not so concerned
about him. But I can't help him read this menu because I forgot my
glasses. Can you leave the lights on or do you have a flashlight?'"

—Risa

Sibling facilitators used the only tools they had, based on speech and lipreading. However, despite good intentions, the tools functioned like Band-Aids, giving the illusion of providing access but for many failed to convey complex ideas to foster siblings from knowing one another at deeper levels. Both deaf and hearing siblings who used sign insisted their learning it at an early age was crucial: their sibling relationships developed through countless signed interactions. Mingling with native users, as children, guarantees both siblings will fully acquire both languages. When we asked the siblings how they came to learn sign, these were several of their answers:

- *I learned sign language as a kid.*
- *We grew up signing all the time.*
- *My mom took us to sign classes when I was little.*
- *When my parents took me and my brother to deaf events, we hung out a lot with deaf kids and their deaf parents.*

As children, four pairs of deaf and hearing siblings grew up signing with one another. Of the four hearing siblings who signed as children, two have remained Signers as adults. Their use of various MCE systems as opposed to using ASL was a handy companion to repair communication breakdowns, a tool used on the spur of the moment. Signing siblings bluntly stated Sign was the key to getting to know their sibling. At times signing siblings were the only person, on a playground or in a store, who knew Sign and English. Automatically, they would jump in to summarize, throw in Signs to clarify, fill in gaps, or interject their thoughts and observations. Using Signs, they had a guarantee deaf siblings would understand, compared to depending on the improbabilities of understanding someone's lip movements, a tool used by the non-signing siblings frozen in oral methods. In addition to using their tool, two languages to convey spoken or sign information, signing siblings readily gave advice. Transparency wasn't feasible: they'd give tips on how to interact with deaf siblings to those who had never met a deaf person before. Deeply invested in the interaction, they needed to do it. How could they ignore or allow others to ignore their deaf sibling? Their mission was accomplished. Deaf and hearing siblings, using sign in everyday lives when they were out and about, gave the deaf siblings visibility, enabling them to participate in family and neighborhood conversations.

The deaf siblings who grew up with hearing siblings who signed were playmates who could function as siblings are supposed to—as socialization agents. Through play, as both deaf and hearing siblings developed social skills, deaf siblings' confidence increased: expressing opinions, learning how ask for things, arguing, sharing possessions and their secret thoughts— the social skills necessary to get along with people. If siblings are struggling to communicate with one another, it adds yet another stumbling block for resolving naturally arising conflicts, a key component of getting along. The fictionalized story "Fish with Thorns" illustrates how naturally siblings interact with one another in sign without the attachment of deaf or hearing attributions.

FISH WITH THORNS

Haley asked, "Hey, Mom, when are you leaving to pick up Terrence at school? I haven't seen him since spring break!"

"On Friday, but don't even think about joining me. I need to talk with Terrence alone."

"Does that mean you will tell him about the divorce?"

"Of course."

"He will be really upset. Please ... I want to go with you so I can be there when you tell him."

"No way. This is a parent's job. You'll see him the minute we get home and will have him for the rest of the summer."

Terrence was packing up the last few items. His roommate was vacuuming the room.

"Hey, Andy, can you help me carry my trunk downstairs? My mom and sister are on their way."

"Sure. I know you told me, but we've been so busy with finals. Tell me again what you're doing for the summer."

"Fishing in the creek and hanging out with my sister, Haley. It's been over six months since I've seen her."

"Oops! I forgot you have a sister. What's she like?"

"She's fun to hang out with, although she can be high-strung. You know, I'm a laid-back kind of guy. Sometimes we clash, but in the end, we get along well."

"Is that your mom's blue van?"

Terrence raced out to the van. As Mom stepped out, Terrence asked: "Hey, Mom, where's Haley? You came alone? Why?"

"Gimme a kiss! I miss you! We'll talk later. Get your things into the van so we can get moving! Hi Andy! Nice seeing you again."

Terrence threw his suitcases into the van and climbed into the front seat. His mom didn't start the van but turned to him. "Give me a minute and I'll explain."

"Mom ... is Haley really okay? What's going on? She always comes with you at the end of the year to pick me up! Come on, tell me! Where is she?"

"OK. OK. I wanted to tell you without Haley here. So here goes...." She took a deep breath. "Dad and I are getting divorced."

"Oh ... you know, I'm not surprised. You and dad didn't really talk to each other much. Right?"

"That pretty much says it all. We just aren't happy together any more. Most important, I want you to understand it is not about you or Haley. It's between me and Dad."

"How did Haley take it?"

"She's extremely upset. She blames it on me. But the truth is it is really both of us. Not just me."

"I know. Several of the kids at school have divorced parents, and they've talked about it. No one is at fault."

Back at the house, Haley was pacing the driveway, dreading but at the same time excited about Terrence's arrival. The minute the van arrived, Terrence jumped out.

Haley hugged Terrence tightly and dragged him into the bedroom. "Did Mom tell you about their divorce?"

"Yeah, Mom says you blame her. Not true!"

"That's BS! You haven't heard them arguing non-stop! Mom started the whole thing. She was the one who told him SHE wanted the divorce."

"I saw you eavesdropping but you brushed me off and you refused to tell me what they were talking about!"

"Come on! I was protecting you! It's awful what they said to each other. You have no idea."

"But I am older than you! You should have told me."

"Leave it alone. We're not discussing this anymore!"

"Can we talk about the divorce? I know it's hard on us, but if you let me, we can deal with it together."

"Look, Terrence, listen to me. I said no, I told you before. I don't want to discuss it."

"OK, Fine. But Jeopardy is coming on in half an hour. Will you watch it with me? I'll bet I can still beat you!" he teased.

"No thanks," she responded glumly. "I'm not in the mood. You'll have to just watch it yourself. You'll get most of the answers. You always do."

"That's not the point. I'd just like to spend some happy time with you, instead of watching you sink into such a funk." But Haley slumped over even further and looked down at her feet.

Terrence spent the rest of the summer trying to approach his sister to talk about the divorce, but she angrily rejected every effort. One day, in exasperation, he called his roommate on the videophone.

"Hey, Andy, how's the summer been for you? Mine wasn't great at all. As you know, my parents are getting divorced and my sister isn't talking to me either!"

"Yikes! That's too bad! I thought you two were tight."

"Yes, but lately, my sister's been like a blowfish, with deadly thorns, stabbing my heart, like that fish we saw in the movie last winter. Like she's lashed out at me, criticizing my girlfriend's clothes and chastising me for eating her ice cream."

"Why not talk with your parents about her?"

"Impossible! Mom and my sister are at odds with each other. Dad is no better because he doesn't sign—we barely understand one another."

The above fictionalized story scratches the surface of the contrasting perspectives of a deaf brother and a hearing Signing sister who were interviewed separately. We are compelled to point out the deaf-hearing issues are uppermost in the discussion with the hearing Signing sister, though barely mentioned by her deaf brother. Haley vented her frustrations with hearing people:

> Most people didn't understand his speech, and I understood his signs better than anyone, so I got to be his voice. I've also had to defend him against strangers and occasionally against relatives who made fun of his voice and his signing. How dare they! I'm always waiting for another injustice to happen.

Growing up, these siblings' parents learned to Sign soon after Terrence became deaf. Since Terrence and Haley were both young, they quickly picked it up, faster than their mom, though each described her as fairly proficient for a second-language learner. His public school taught them Signed English, and it worked well enough. Eventually, Terrence learned ASL at the residential school, but he was always willing to switch back to Signed English for his sister and mom.

Everywhere these siblings went, Terrence and Haley both knew Haley was always watching out for him, was there for him, always willing to defend him. Even though Terrence trusts her more than anyone else, which she didn't mind at all, he is baffled: *"Why can't she let me be there for her, just this once? There must be a way, but I sure haven't been able to find it."* If we look at Terrence's response to Haley from the perspective of an older sibling trying to console a younger one, then Terrence's being deaf and Haley's hearing is irrelevant to conflict in the story. Although shared language allowed them to communicate effortlessly, it was not a guarantee of a stress-free relationship. On Cicirelli and Gold's continuum, their relationship probably falls somewhere between Loyal and Congenial. The difficulties they faced in this situation will not change their long-lasting close relationship. The divorce was a trigger for Terrence to seize the opportunity to exchange his role from being the protected and taken-care-of sibling to being the one to provide support. In many families, role reversals occur more often than we expect. As individuals face challenges, they try on different roles and try to break long-established patterns. It seems Haley wasn't ready to surrender her habitual caretaking role, but Terrence has laid the foundation for a change in their future relationship.

Since siblings' relationships are interdependent, these deaf and hearing siblings' Sign communication made it possible to have natural spontaneity most siblings have with one another. Larry, Judy's older brother, didn't have the luxury of signing with his sisters. In retrospect, he realized how suffocating his childhood had been:

> Upon discovering how much easier sign language was, as I acquired deaf friends, I became aware of give and take that was lacking with oral communication. Although still close, my relationship with Mary Ann changed. With Judy picking up sign language, our relationship blossomed.

Unlike Larry and Judy, growing up with a sibling who Signed was all siblings like Terrence and Haley knew, until deaf friends from school told them about sisters or brothers who didn't sign. Deaf siblings never had given a moment's thought to how different their lives would have been if their sibling didn't sign. One deaf sibling, Randall, was shocked and distressed: "*Whoa. I was thinking to myself, 'If it was me, it would be really difficult for me to imagine that.'*" He reported that several friends had told him, "*I wish my sister could be like that.*" Some siblings were horrified to see their deaf friends trapped in hearing families with no place to vent, realizing the discussions they had engaged in at home with family members who signed, gave them the conversational experience to provide emotional support to their deaf friends. Equally important, signing siblings contributed to deaf siblings' social development. Like dropping a pebble into a lake, the social skills learned through their signing siblings had repercussions far beyond the immediate family, spilling into the DEAF-WORLD, invigorating it.

Tools of repairing communication breakdowns and providing tips for engaging in conversations with a deaf sibling were not only for casual acquaintances; they permeated family events too. Signing siblings conveyed Dad's political commentary, Grandma describing her dreadful appendix attack, or a deaf sibling's vacation plans to exotic places. However, as deaf siblings approached adolescence, they saw how quickly they were surpassing hearing siblings in ASL. With peers in school and deaf adults at social events, deaf siblings became skilled users of ASL, discarding Sign they used in school and with their hearing families. Kevin commented about the impact on his hearing sister: "*I had moved on with learning ASL and finding it my language. ASL is really me. My sister only had Signed English, which left her behind.*"

When Signing siblings realized that MCE systems were limiting interactions with their deaf siblings, they realized proficiency in ASL was a lifelong undertaking. Even as adults, several worried whether they signed correctly, expressing concern about forming the hand shapes, holding the palm in the right direction or putting fingertips on the right places on the body. Learning new vocabulary and putting facial expressions in alignment with emotions was a constant challenge each time Signing siblings conversed with deaf people. Missing the ASL nuances of grammar or the subject or object, Signing siblings often didn't understand whether an event had happened or would happen or who did what to whom. Imagine Signing siblings as individuals who studied Spanish but never lived in a Spanish-speaking country. The Signing siblings suddenly discovered their level of language competence had reached a plateau, which is best described by Mahshie:

> (Cummins 1991) has identified a very important distinction in levels of language competence in bilingual speakers: basic interpersonal communication skills (BICS) and cognitive academic language proficiency (CALP). BICS is the level of language performance, which is sufficient for face-to-face interaction, where the speaker can rely heavily on context, and the content is often somewhat predictable [S. Mahshie 1997, 8].

To their mutual dismay these siblings, hearing and deaf, found themselves simultaneously accelerating on different levels in the two languages they were acquiring, English and ASL. The hearing siblings' knowledge base had moved onto the CALP level, but their Sign skills remained at a BICS level. Simultaneously, the deaf siblings' signing had leaped from BICS to CALP, but according to hearing siblings, some of deaf siblings' English knowledge base was not moving at the same pace.

These multidimensional aspects have amplified how and why Signing siblings were feeling limited in their ability to understand deaf siblings. Initially, signing siblings became acutely aware they did not share the same knowledge base as their deaf siblings, instinctively realizing how they absorbed voluminous amounts of information by osmosis from eavesdropping on conversations as well as radio, television and other media. As they entered their teens, they were shocked and appalled at the amount of incidental information their deaf siblings did *not* pick up.

At one of many family poker games, Newman recalled family members' disbelief their deaf brother had played hours of poker but did not fully grasp all the rules. Though he came in third, "*he just didn't know something as simple ... he didn't understand what a straight was or he didn't know you could have a full house.*" The false assumption was that everyone started with the same poker knowledge base, on an equal footing with other players. However, the hearing brother's illusion was destined to create a distance between the brothers. In fact, the hearing brother was ignorant and appeared to be unaware that his deaf brother did not acquire information if it was solely available through sound. Although the deaf sibling could have learned the rules from the Internet or from playing with deaf friends who might have explained the varieties of winning hands, the fact remains he played the game based on partial knowledge.

Another facet contributing to the lack of common ground was the deaf siblings' progression in language acquisition. Some deaf siblings arrived at school with no language; one didn't even know she had a name. Others began with spoken language training, and eventually used MCE systems in mainstreamed settings. The tipping point in the sibling relations was deaf siblings' exposure to ASL in their teens, when they began to use the language extensively to socialize with deaf peers. Several Signing siblings probably wondered: "Who was this stranger who used to be my playmate and friend?" For the first time, they saw how deaf siblings defended their beliefs, argued their case, expressed opinions and negotiated with friends or teachers in ways they had not done before using speech or MCE systems. In addition, these Signing siblings were hypnotized by how deaf siblings were into give-and-take conversations with deaf peers, with no mental energy expended to understand the words or the concepts. Although they had worked out an adequate way of communicating with their deaf sibling, Signing siblings conceded it had been an ongoing struggle, an indefinable something else was always lurking. As they watched deaf siblings' effortless interactions with deaf friends, they saw that ASL, the language itself, was the key ingredient.

Three siblings' lives are forever transformed by one sister's decision to learn Sign in this fictionalized story, "A Tight Threesome." Witnessing her other family members having in-depth conversations with their deaf brother, she is determined not to continue to have stagnating, limited, superficial interactions with him.

A TIGHT THREESOME

Nadia, the eldest of three siblings, was out of the house when her deaf brother Rory graduated from his Oral elementary school, and transferred to a deaf residential school, where he acquired ASL. The youngest sister, Val, eagerly looked forward to her deaf brother coming home on weekends and holidays. Spending time with him, she was immersed in ASL. In his late teens, Rory's vision began to deteriorate, starting with tunnel vision. He was told he had Usher's syndrome. Both sisters completed college, were married and had careers, while Rory was still living at home with their parents.

NADIA CALLED VAL: "Hey sis, what are we gonna do about Rory? He'll have to live with one of us."

VAL: "No way! He can take care of himself. I've seen many deaf-blind people like him do just fine living independently."

NADIA: "How is this possible? Mom does everything for him—the laundry, cooking. I don't even know if he's contributing anything towards household expenses."

VAL: "Of course he has been! But he needs his own apartment. Our parents aren't getting any younger and can't do this much longer. We can help him find one but he'd have to find a roommate to share the expenses. We must talk with him and do it ASAP."

NADIA: "OK, sis. You're the one who has the best communication with Rory. I've always felt incompetent and awkward interacting with him. I'm getting better with my Signs, but have a long way to go."

VAL: "You sure have improved! I remember when you first took ASL classes. You know, for a while Rory and I were resistant and felt uneasy since we had our own private conversations. It was sorta like you were invading our territory. But then I realized that instead of seeing you as someone who usurped my interpreting role, I was actually relieved and grateful that you finally have your own relationship with Rory."

NADIA: "I know. I felt it. But thank goodness, we're over that. I do the best I can, though I'll never match your magnificent ASL. You know, you and Rory get a kick out of spelling and signing into one another's hands and then you burst out laughing. I envy your proficiency—c'est la vie. So you talk with Rory about getting his own place. OK?"

VAL: "Fair enough. I'll bring it up with him. I'm not so sure of his feelings, but I think he'll be receptive to this idea. But I have to know I have your support behind me and that you'll talk with him too, reinforcing what I've told him. Either of us can go with him to find an apartment."

NADIA: "Right, and I know he tends to be patient with me, though I'm always nervous when I'm Signing. And he has plenty of deaf friends. You never know who else could use a roommate. Rory earns enough and can afford the rent."

Nadia changed and brought the three siblings closer than ever. In the above story, she broke their family patterns by being proactive, taking ASL classes so she could put an end to her superficial interactions with Rory. She adamantly told Judy: *"Families take care of one another. That's what we do."* Taking care of one another also implies doing something that requires a sibling to make herself available and accessible to another sibling.

Despite their limitations in ASL, Signing siblings like Val and Nadia were steadfast, ready and willing to use Sign interacting with clerks, postal workers, and relatives who often became paralyzed when confronted with their deaf sibling. Deaf siblings like Rory and Terrence described themselves as being tolerant, sensitive and patient by naturally and willingly adjusting their signing to match their signing siblings' emerging ASL skills. Both deaf and hearing siblings saw sign as their prized possession, in contrast to many deaf friends whose siblings did not. Getting siblings to converse with one another sufficiently, respectfully dealing with one another's language limitations, was a step closer to having insider's knowledge of each other's lives as people.

12

Sibling-Interpreters

"It was just normal to me. No big deal. He was just my brother who happened to be deaf."—Judy

Several hearing siblings we interviewed talked about their dual roles as family interpreter and as professional interpreters. Their fluency in ASL and English, and familiarity with deaf and hearing cultures, allowed them to comfortably immerse themselves in these coexisting entities. Meanwhile, deaf siblings saw their sibling-interpreters as siblings first in spite of these dual roles. Yet these dual roles often led the hearing siblings into primal struggles which, for the most part, they kept to themselves. Golda, talking about her feelings towards her deaf sister, put it this way: *"I want you to be a part of what's going on, more than I care about the fact that I have to interpret...."* Several hearing siblings expressed similar thoughts, setting the tone for why they interpret. However, the experience in their practical lives—as adults—barely shows the anguish. Every day, deaf and hearing siblings encountered people who were oblivious about how to interact with a deaf person. Even though both siblings were acutely aware of the deaf sibling's isolation, these sibling-interpreters took it upon themselves to relieve the tensions caused by these encounters. They interpreted spontaneously when out and about with deaf siblings: on the beach, at a restaurant, at an airport or in a store. In these settings, often the personal experiences as hearing siblings undermined their professional interpreter roles. Sibling-interpreters felt the agony of being inconspicuous, taken for granted and neglected by everyone except the deaf sibling, yet both deaf and hearing siblings knew the contribution was immeasurable. In return, deaf siblings have expressed fear about the potential consequences of their hearing siblings' interpreting.

Although intense involvement inevitably came with risks of imminent power in their everyday lives, sibling-interpreters still see their role as a bridge. They would facilitate communication *until* deaf siblings and hearing family members had their own relationships with one another: at family meals, gatherings of neighbors, friends, relatives, schools, stores, or any time they are together. Contrary to their hands-on experiences, these sibling professionals felt the national professional organization was breathing down their necks. The Registry of Interpreters for the Deaf (RID) sets the standards for working interpreters, with a Code of Professional Conduct (CPC) for ethical behavior (Code of Professional Conduct n.d.). These deaf and hearing siblings took issue with the profession, which implied that sibling-interpreters should "not interpret for their family members." As children, hearing siblings began as Signers, soaking up vocabulary like sponges to communicate as playmates and to include their deaf sibling whenever the circumstances warranted. However, as adults, as hearing siblings made the transition to interpreters, they hadn't anticipated its innumerable ramifications. During professional training, sibling-interpreters analyzed the linguistic features of ASL, examined the interpreting process and its ethical considerations, and studied deaf history in the context of an oppressed minority. In addition, Deaf Arts (ASL Literature, ASL poetry, Deaf theater) enriched their lives, providing insights into how the DEAF-WORLD, with its own language and culture, formed a community—one that became their second family. As the hearing siblings became more knowledgeable about the DEAF-WORLD, they were baffled and appalled that they had the privilege of studying ASL and deaf history, while most of the deaf people they worked with, as well as their own siblings, were rarely given the opportunity.

In spite of the injustice deaf and hearing siblings experienced daily, unconscious dynamics emerged as hearing siblings worked in the hearing world, camouflaging their roles as professional interpreters. Unsettled feelings arose as little voices reminding them: their professional and personal lives were inextricably intertwined. At home, sibling-interpreters felt good being the designated family interpreter, a prestigious status the family had granted by some unspoken agreement, presumably based on firsthand knowledge of the deaf sibling's history, quirks and mannerisms. Succinctly, one hearing sibling, Shari, expressed the thoughts of several others when she said: "*I just assumed interpreting was part of my childhood and because I knew him best, I should be the one doing it.*"

No one in the family had ever discussed their role as the interpreters. It evolved as they stumbled along, learning through trial and error, with deaf siblings feeding them Signs and trusting them as their voices. However, as sibling-interpreters felt at home in their new profession, apprehension appeared with an admonishing tone: "You can't be neutral." Instantly, these hearing sibling-interpreters dismissed the warning: "This is different. She's my sister! I can't sit idly by and ignore her puzzled look, asking me what the dentist just said."

In the family environment, even though they had deaf siblings' tacit approval, sibling-interpreters realized that, by participating in deaf siblings' conversations as an interpreter, they were privy to personal interests, gossip, political agendas, and other tidbits of information about their deaf sibling and the hearing person. Yet they were hammered by these thoughts:

- What did Aunt Amanda just say that was so rude? I'm not going to let her get away with this. I gotta talk to my sister about this!
- I can't stand how patronizing Grandpa was to my sister. Why do I have to interpret this?
- I need to take care of my daughter but I see Uncle Jeff and my brother's conversation is falling apart!

Despite conflicting forces that shook their equilibrium, sibling-interpreters continued to interpret, alternating between being a playmate, confidante, or rival one moment, and switching into interpreter persona the next. In one sense it was an honor to have access to their deaf siblings' interactions. On the other hand, it was a tremendous responsibility. Sometimes they admitted they would learn things about their deaf sibling they'd rather not have known about, though their deaf siblings didn't seem to mind. To these deaf siblings, access outweighed the privacy issues. In the family setting, the sibling-interpreters never knew when they'd have to resist a knee-jerk reaction to add a suggestion, opinion or disagreement. In their minds, they heard their colleagues' reprimand, "You're overstepping the neutral boundaries you pledged to respect." As sibling-interpreters like Judy slipped in and out of dual roles with their deaf sibling, her inner voice may have supported their bias:

> How could I not be a participant when our families have grown to include spouses, children and other extended relatives who have no experience interacting with deaf people and don't sign? This is family! Since no one seems to mind, why should I?

Sometimes it mattered to a family member. When it happens, compromises are typically made for the sake of peace in the family, even if access is compromised.

> At one of our family celebrations, my sister-in-law Carolyn warned me of my sister's anger while I was interpreting. Mary Ann was used to having direct eye contact with Larry, but he was looking at me. Until that moment, I never realized I had usurped Mary Ann's role in the family. Her face and body language were loud and clear: She resented my presence. I needed to get out of their conversations. And I did.

Jumping In

Similar to Judy's experience, the more these sibling-interpreters learned about the formal interpreting process, the more they realized the family interpreting they had done all their lives was different: it was unplanned, reflexive and unexpected. As far as we know, the deaf and hearing siblings never considered it as a topic even needing to be discussed: it was spontaneous. In contrast, in their professional roles the sibling-interpreters were ravenous researchers, repositories of knowledge, never knowing whether they would be sent to a hospital, parent-teacher conference, art museum, a funeral or any location where deaf and hearing people interact. In addition, they would convey whatever transpired between the deaf and hearing participants. Quality interpreting required understanding the intentions of the participants: it could be information sharing, an altercation or pitches made by a salesperson. Sibling-interpreters were always in the moment. Research in a family setting was superfluous; they already had an encyclopedia of insider's knowledge about their deaf sibling and the hearing people involved, mostly relatives and family friends. Whenever one or the other thought interpreting might be necessary, conversations between deaf and hearing siblings often began with a questioning eye glance and a head nod followed by a wordless negotiation, totally aware of their synchronicity, making instant decisions on the spur of moment whether or not the hearing sibling was to interpret.

From a lifetime of making spontaneous decisions, passion enriched the sibling-interpreter's professional work. Living with a deaf sibling, they internalized this belief: deaf people deserved the chance to do all the things people do to convey thoughts and emotions to fellow human beings. Sibling-interpreters' access attitudes were meticulous yet principled about "deaf rights": ASL, Bilingual-Bicultural education, accessibility, and interpreting. However, when it came to family, it was impossible to leave their private lives at home and remain unbiased. Being with their deaf sibling was, by definition, an event comprising a lifetime of irreplaceable sibling connections defying neutrality. Deaf and hearing siblings—like all siblings—grew up together, had intimate knowledge of each other's foibles, idiosyncrasies, vulnerabilities and strengths. They had honed each other's interests or skills, negotiated their needs within the family, and been lifelong companions. Together, as siblings, they had shared deep emotionally laden events: the birth of another sibling, the death of a grandparent or the joy of a Bat Mitzvah celebration. Emotional connections are formed early, but the professional undercurrents for unconscious and later the conscious behaviors telling sibling-interpreters what they should and should not do, kept nagging at them. They were to "Refrain from providing counsel, advice, or personal opinions" and "decline assignments or withdraw from the interpreting profession when not competent due to physical, mental or emotional factors" (Code of Professional Conduct n.d.). Some sibling-interpreters felt alone, on the fence, not knowing what to do, possibly leaving the deaf sibling even more isolated. The only people deaf and hearing siblings knew of who could relate best to these experiences were hearing children of deaf adults—codas—some of whom were also chosen as their designated family interpreters.

Spontaneous interpreting by sibling-interpreters throughout their adult lives symbolizes ardent perseverance to do everything possible to involve deaf siblings in their surroundings. Irrefutably, the hearing siblings held a distinct advantage over deaf siblings: firsthand access to auditory information. They heard nuances of verbal innuendos, where the tone of voice was integral to creating the mood. Sibling-interpreters were also tuned into environmental sounds like a baby crying, a plane overhead, or a door slamming, all of which contribute to the energy and liveliness of social gatherings. Each time sibling-interpreters shared this integral information, it gave their deaf siblings the latitude to decide whether they were distractions or not.

At a family picnic, while sibling-interpreters are busy setting the table, overhearing a squabble between relatives or picking up an upcoming celebration, they begin to wonder whether to interpret the surrounding buzz. They have to decide, but it's always a balancing act, juggling between "what I want" versus "what I think my deaf sibling wants." They might choose to do nothing, at the moment, but save what they heard for a later email, text message or videophone chat. Or was what they heard so juicy the designated family interpreter should steal her deaf sister's attention and begin interpreting? The sibling-interpreter may know, from an argument they had the previous week, the topic is a pet peeve of her deaf sibling who would salivate to butt in with her viewpoints. Late-night exchanges bring intimacy at family gatherings. Judy illustrates such an opportunity in the life of being a hearing sibling with a deaf brother:

> As soon as we sent the interpreter on her way, after my husband's birthday celebration, it was way past 11:00 p.m. but several of our adult children, along with a few of our sister's children, were schmoozing in the family room. There I was, sitting adjacent to everyone, engrossed in sign, with my deaf brother and sister-in-law. Suddenly my ears perked up, I stopped signing and held my hand signaling "hold on," and turned my head to eavesdrop. "My gosh," I signed, "they are talking about the money Uncle Leonard lost in the stock market!" Before I had a chance to ask if they wanted to finish up our conversation, without a moment's hesitation, we found ourselves in the circle and I began interpreting.

Every interpreted interaction gave these sibling pairs topics about a relative to mull over later, tidbits about shared events for future discussions, or perhaps vacation sites to consider because the sibling pair heard about them from a favorite cousin. Meanwhile, deaf siblings who grew up with sibling-interpreters say they "take in all they can," seeing it as part of their sibling experience. Sibling-interpreters' on-the-spot decisions were propelled by the depth of an alliance with deaf siblings, coupled with the belief their deaf siblings were entitled to mingle to whatever extent possible.

The Alliance

Professional interpreters self-monitor their interpretations, making sure they've conveyed the intentions and all speakers' nuanced discourse between people who don't know each other's language. Unlike the reactive aspect of interpreters to their work, sibling monitoring is proactive, a result of the emotional investment individuals have in their deaf siblings and the insights they have, precisely because they are family, not an employee. An interpreter strives to be neutral; siblings are connatural with one another. A recent description of an interpreter in an educational setting describes the type of monitor hearing siblings can be to deaf siblings:

> I want to be inside their minds. This becomes a very intimate partnership.... I can also watch what the eyes of the deaf and the hard of hearing students are seeing.... I am "eye-activated." If a student looks at me, I sign. When eyes are busy elsewhere, I alternate between noticing what they are looking at and also watching and trying to understand what the teacher is showing.... I am also listening very carefully to the teacher's words and inflection for content that is not being shown; that is, anything that the deaf and hard of hearing students are NOT seeing. I signal the students in overt or in subtle ways, inviting them to give me their attention and then sign what I have heard that they did not see.... I learned something invaluable by watching them [Rodman 2011, 36–37].

As the interpreter described here, during monitoring, many thoughts race through the hearing sibling-interpreters' minds. If they spot a misunderstanding, confusion, cultural gap or cue from their deaf sibling, unlike the interpreter in the classroom who is paid to be available, as siblings they have choices: whether or not to offer assistance, give up what they're doing, or do nothing. Regardless of the decision while they are monitoring, similar to sibling facilitators and signing siblings, they are rarely relaxed.

Despite the power imbalance, with hearing siblings having the upper hand of being the first to know, the sibling-interpreters we interviewed echoed one another as they described their relationship with their deaf sibling:

PEARL: He's my best friend.
BREE: My sister and I are very close.

Each time they witnessed and refused to be part of deaf siblings' unrelenting isolation, sibling-interpreters stood fast as the designated family interpreter. What's more, they held dearly to an unequivocal belief in communication access, and out of necessity tuned out the negative undercurrents of colleagues to achieve an ultimate goal: to be engaged in each other's lives not only as siblings but as lifetime friends. Keenly aware of their hearing status advantage, the sibling-interpreters came to treasure the gift they had acquired: ASL and interpreting skills as tools, fostering intimacy with their deaf sibling.

These sibling-interpreters and their deaf counterparts have a partnership they both cherish. Cicirelli and Gold's continuum defines the intensity of their adult sibling relationships, somewhere between:

> **The Intimate**—they are especially close and extremely devoted. They valued their relationship above all others and
> **The Congenial**—they feel they are friends. They are close and caring but place a higher value on their own marriages and parent-child relationships.

As peers from childhood to adulthood, these deaf and hearing siblings' relationship have evolved as they matured. The placement on Cicirelli and Gold's intensity continuum, indicating how close the siblings felt towards one another, was a result of the hearing sibling-interpreters' awareness and sensitivity to their deaf sibling's isolation. Every encounter in the hearing world taught resilience. The deaf siblings inevitably brought that resiliency to the ups and downs of their sibling relationship. In return, several hearing siblings who became professional interpreters believed their immersion in the DEAF-WORLD was a gift, leading to fulfilling, rewarding careers.

Interpreting between languages and cultures goes to the heart of creating human connection and communication. Learning the language is different from learning to interpret. To be bilingual—mastering dual languages—is necessary but isn't sufficient to be an interpreter. Another skill layer is added. You are conscious of a constant interaction going on between people of different languages and cultures which test your cultural competency: it becomes emotionally gratifying, intellectually stimulating and challenging. One sibling, Golda, explains vividly the transformation, almost spiritually:

> I feel very blessed to be in the DEAF-WORLD and I also realized that if I didn't have my sister who was deaf, I wouldn't be as involved to the extent that I'm involved. My sister really changed my life ... she helps me look at the world in a very different way. I think that my perspective is much broader and my eyes are much more in tune to body language, what people are saying and what they look like.

On the other hand, when Judy asked the hearing siblings: "Why didn't you learn to sign?" they were instantly on guard, knowing their deaf siblings wished they signed. Arguably in their defense, Trish made a valid point which was almost convincing: *"But you've also chosen to embrace his world and make it your life, your profession."* For those who used sign, years of childhood play fostered interactions, thus nurturing the ever-increasing sign and interpreting skills of the hearing siblings. In addition, numerous sorts of conversations have infused these siblings with acceptance and love to thrive in respective roles as siblings who are lifelong peers and confidants.

Rewards have granted both deaf and hearing siblings the opportunity to see many dimensions of the two communities they inhabit—keeping them grounded with reality—many aspects of the daily life they might not have been aware existed. It isn't a job, but a career that some hearing siblings have chosen, to embrace love for ASL, deaf people, and exposure to a variety of experiences, which they call an exploration of life. The rewards of giving turned up in little niches in their work, each time they interpreted for deaf people they knew from the community or had never met. Their passion and compassion were showered with praise, gratitude and words of encouragement but weren't picture-perfect either. Anxiety came with the job: how to enter one's comfort zone with deaf and hearing consumers and search for what each wanted, assess skills and emotions, and educate people how to effectively use ASL interpreters. In addition was the constant challenge of witnessing audism and oppression and dealing with the aftermath of the stress it caused. Notwithstanding doubts, Val recalls how her family saw the pride she took in choosing to do community interpreting work. *"My deaf brother's very, very proud, my sister too, and my husband's so excited. They all love the fact that I'm an interpreter. It's just so different in itself, and so I'm really grateful."*

Not everyone gets to grow up with deaf siblings; it's a rare phenomenon. But to the sibling-interpreters it was second nature. They instinctively bridged cultural gaps each time situations arose to address and diffuse awkward moments—like when a hearing person got flustered at a first encounter with their deaf sibling. The fringe benefit of earning a living, that began as the family's designated volunteer and grew into being a professional interpreter, was deeply rooted in affection and respect for their deaf sibling. Bree put it this way: *"She really gave me the language ... brought information back to her about the hearing world and I learned about the deaf world through her."* What started in childhood continued throughout their lives, sharing news of people they knew even in different states, controversial issues affecting deaf people's lives, deaf events, and politics in the DEAF-WORLD, a never-ending source of mutual interest.

Interpreter-siblings like Bree in "Tell Me What You Hear" or the two sisters in "A Tight Threesome" have another potent tool: they form an alliance with their deaf sibling, so neither has to bear the emotional burden of being alone in their own isolation as siblings. They have one another as sounding boards rather than holding everything inside, where feelings rot and fester. No further discussions were needed. These two were in sync, empathetic towards one another, not having to wonder if the other was feeling any differently. In the alliance bubble, an immediate safe haven, they do reality checks of their frustrations, balance out their points of view and clarify the many cultural-behavior misunderstandings that occur during deaf and hearing interactions, especially with non-signing relatives or family friends. They brainstorm strategies for upcoming events. The bubble is an island of their own, to hone problem-solving skills and test the waters for observations, knowing the other is not there to judge but help them grow. Deaf and hearing siblings, as partners, develop competent skills in areas of networking, negotiation, social media literacy and effective communication skills to meet the demands of complex American society.

Hiring Outsiders

Another essential issue hearing and deaf siblings had to contend with, in the bubble, surrounds hiring ASL interpreters for family events. In general, families tended to hire interpreters they know, either from the deaf sibling's school, work or local community events. Various family members took on responsibility for contacting interpreters and arranging payment. Typically, hiring interpreters was based on an underlying belief that the interpreters are hired for the deaf person, like a ramp provides means of entry only for a person in a wheelchair. Sibling-interpreters experienced the adverse reactions of their families as well as other non-signing people. Hearing parents, siblings, and relatives were unprepared, not fully understanding why suddenly ASL interpreters were at family events when all their lives, they felt "we did just fine." The sibling-interpreter, however, felt differently; an interpreter was just one of many tools available to facilitate communication. In spite of negative feelings toward non-signers, sibling-interpreters, in general, were comfortable with the physical presence of an outsider. Nor did they share the discomfort of other family members who behaved awkwardly with the stranger in their midst.

Some felt bitter about hiring outsider interpreters at family events. The implication, "My family can't communicate with the deaf family member," caused discomfort. However, the siblings had to bite the bullet and get beyond the embarrassment: the majority of people at these events *were* non-signers. To get to know one's sibling in a different context, such as formal family events where large groups of relatives and/or friends were present, was a luxury most of the siblings we met rarely experienced. In spite of knowing that hiring an interpreter once in a while at a formal family gathering was a benefit serving as temporary relief, families rarely did it.

Deaf siblings saw their hearing siblings happily chatting away with relatives, able to pick up where they left off, at the last gathering or phone call. The deaf siblings and hearing sibling-interpreters were despondent, knowing an interpreter could never make up for the lost years. The deaf siblings admitted to their hearing sibling-interpreters how they envied them. Even with an interpreter, lack of history about the relatives was overwhelming, nor had they had anything in common to chat about. The relatives at family gatherings, especially the non-signing siblings, were totally unaware of the deaf sibling and the sibling-interpreters' bubble-talk. Only the insiders knew it was merely an illusion that hiring interpreters would alleviate the pain of isolation. Siblings typically keep each other informed of family gossip. However, deaf siblings did not have the information to share or to reflect upon when they got home. With only erratic instances of hiring interpreters, they rarely were able to stay updated with knowing the hobbies, interests, etc., of who these people were, how they were connected to one another, or much about them. Yet deaf siblings knew there was more to these relationships than the superficialities they were experiencing.

Furthermore, the illusion of a safety net, hiring an interpreter, sends a message: hearing relatives, including non-signing siblings, are off the hook. Rarely did anyone in the family insist or urge them to learn ASL. Despair was evident when deaf siblings suddenly realized their hearing siblings had an instant ticket to family membership but they did not.

Hiring interpreters for family events is not a panacea allowing relationships to flourish, but it serves as a beginning tool. Ideally, every family could return to Martha's Vineyard, an island inhabited by the largest documented population of deaf people from the 17th century until the middle of the 20th century (Groce and Whiting 1985). They were a visibly blended community where the majority of residents used sign language. Years later, as researchers came to study the phenomenon, they were astonished to learn that the former residents interviewed didn't have any inkling who was deaf or hearing. Twenty-first-century equivalents of Martha's Vineyard exist in other parts of the world: Bedouins in Israel and Benglaka (Northern Bali, Indonesia). Both areas contain many generations of deaf villagers using forms of communication that have recently been identified as emerging languages to be added to the community of world languages (Solomon 2012).

Whenever families get together, they find ways to communicate. The available tool of hiring an interpreter not only helps families, but also relieves the burden on sibling-interpreters: the chance to socialize, feel secure deaf family members have access to non-signers, and feel elated when non-signing family members take advantage of the opportunity to use the interpreter to chat with deaf relatives. Simultaneously, sibling-interpreters instinctively know its drawbacks do not negate the tool but serve as a buyer beware: An interpreter is a third party in the conversations with non-signing family members, thereby not providing opportunities for experiencing private and direct conversations. As a consequence of the history of fragmented relationships, often the deaf family members and the hired interpreter segregate themselves naturally at family gatherings, yakking the hours away. Regardless of being non-family members to one another, the magnet is the shared language and the DEAF-WORLD.

Deaf siblings and sibling-interpreters who venture in and out of the DEAF-WORLD are no strangers to hiring interpreters for formal family occasions. However, intimate family gatherings force sibling pairs to confront a host of anxieties. Picture a weekend at Grandma's house, way out in a rural area, where a deaf sibling is the only deaf person attending, and the sibling-interpreter has traditionally been the designated family interpreter. Apprehensiveness begins with even introducing the idea of hiring an outside interpreter, knowing they will face inevitable resistance from non-signing relatives used to the status quo. Foremost is persuading relatives why the sibling-interpreter deserved to be off-duty—to be relieved of a non-stop interpreting hell weekend. Selecting an interpreter the entire family would trust with family drama is an additional stress. Another battle would be the inevitable financial responsibility. Who would pick up the tab? Sometimes when frustrations mount, people yearn for change. Rocking the boat is quite intimidating for those trying to effect change and threatening to the affected. Relationships are built on years of social interplay. To challenge the status quo is risky, especially when you're confronting people you love: your parents and extended family of grandparents, aunts, uncles and other relatives who are used to the way things are.

Nevertheless, sometimes sibling-interpreters rock the boat to protect themselves. Often the feeling of threat revolves around personal space and a desire to stay in their comfort zone rather than do what family members impose. One of the major features of dysfunctional families is "the consistent violation of boundaries by the intrusion of family members into functions that are the domains of other family members" (Seligman and Darling 1997, 256). Alma's voice trembled as she relived a painful experience where two boundaries were violated: respect for the hearing sibling's religious beliefs or lack thereof, and recognition of her need to be a sibling at Grandma's house, instead of the designated family interpreter:

> At my grandparents' house, as a teenager, I was interpreting for every meal, for every prayer, even though my immediate family doesn't pray. I didn't know prayer very well, but I had to interpret prayer because that's what my grandparents do. We respected that and went along with it but I always hated it. One time when my aunt asked me to interpret prayer, I just couldn't take it any more so the next time she came over I took her aside and I said, "I'm not comfortable signing the prayer. If you want to do prayer, sign it yourself." And she said, "I don't know how to sign it." And I said, "Try your best."

Alma was fortunate to have found the courage to confront her aunt, yet how did it affect her relationship with her deaf sibling? The conversation between Alma and her aunt did not include her deaf sister. Access became a moot issue since the conflict between the aunt and Alma was at the breaking point. When the interpreting responsibility was thrown to the aunt, her sister's trust in Alma being there for her may have been diminished. Long-term consequences depend on the frequency of these occurrences and whether the siblings take the time to have private conversations, in their bubble, which tends to occur after the fact.

At the time of this event, Alma, two years younger than her sister, was a valiant teenager with minimal religious experience. Yet even as a teenager, she instinctively knew her lack of familiarity with religious material was the key element in her discomfort. The general consensus among experienced professional interpreters is religious interpreting requires ability to understand ancient languages, texts, and multiple references to biblical events as well as the contexts and customs involved in religious settings. Her breaking point was the realization that spontaneous religious interpreting was way over her head. This sibling-interpreter gambled and was willing to accept the potential uproar from the matriarchs in her family. Alma's refusal to interpret was the change agent, causing a ripple effect, affecting everyone in her family, especially the deaf sibling who ultimately is on her own. Other sibling-interpreters shared moments of rocking the boat ranging from taking the power from a relative by being the first to tell a story or even refusing to attend the family gathering, not wanting to be stuck with non-stop interpreting and feeling invisible.

Sometimes extended family members, who are oblivious to years of family patterns, trigger a change in family dynamics, especially with regard to a family's expectations of a designated interpreter, like Judy:

> One day, we all attended a cousin's wedding. To my astonishment, she had hired an interpreter. Voila! I realized someone else could fill those shoes. Shortly after that, my brother, sister and I agreed to split the costs for hiring outside professional interpreters, not only for weddings, funerals and our fifty-people Passover seders, but at our informal birthday parties or BBQs as well. To assure quality interpretation, whoever hosted the event would seek the endorsement or advice

from my deaf brother, his deaf son or me in the selection and hiring of interpreters. Eventually, several of the next generation learned sufficient signs to communicate with our deaf relatives on their own, without an interpreter or me! It was only recently, after our sister passed away, we turned the responsibilities over to the next generation. The family established an Interpreter Fund to which all would contribute, to cover interpreter costs at our families' frequent get-togethers.

The Interpreter Fund passes on to the next generation not only the fiscal responsibility but the knowledge of justice, self-awareness of one's privileges, acceptance of differences, and the value of every family member's determination to be a participating member.[1]

A Family Matter

Throughout our lives, every interaction with our siblings, as children or adults, adds to our wealth of knowledge about them, helping us to know them better. These interactions have the potential to bring us closer or to divide us. Sometimes interactions backfire, especially in families where relationships are tentative or distant, disclosing how little siblings actually know one another. Since Marla and her siblings are rarely in contact with one another, family gatherings tend to center around life-cycle events, where traditionally an interpreter has been hired. However, assumptions and misunderstandings continue their vicious cycle, making harmony elusive:

> At any upcoming family event, I always dreaded having to bring up the discussion about hiring interpreters with my siblings. Even though we rarely discussed the logistics, our mother always picked up the tab, relieving us all of any acknowledgment that access is a family matter.

Was there a way for conversations to take place where opportunities for exchanging ideas could be conducted? Why was the conversation limited to Marla and her mom? In most of the families we interviewed, parents picked up the tab for hiring ASL interpreters at large gatherings. Patterns don't change easily. Deaf and hearing siblings saw how their parents paid for speech lessons, hearing aids and interpreters during their childhood days, and it just continues despite the fact siblings are adults. Discussing money matters is a sore subject for any family, especially when in reality access is expensive and can be a burden to one person. Paying for interpreters is much more efficient as a family matter than as any one individual's taking on the sole responsibility. Interpreters are costly, so it's an easy task to spread the costs among many users.

In addition, since siblings were not involved when their parents paid for these deaf-related things, family patterns take over. Siblings have no reason to think they are part of it, unless someone raises the issue—wants to break the pattern or rock the boat. Often, it begins with getting the support from those who are not dependent upon the access. The fact remains hiring interpreters *is* a family matter. It is a beginning step to foster conversations where access is in everyone's interest including the next generation of nieces and nephews who could benefit from a conversation with a deaf aunt or uncle, with the tool of an interpreter to perhaps break the ice. Since hearing family members are outsiders to the DEAF-WORLD, if they become engaged in conversations with deaf family members, they may learn about the complexities involved in hiring an ASL interpreter.

Securing funding for hiring interpreters is always a challenge. However, other than setting up Family Interpreter Funds, families have addressed the issue in alternative ways: sibling-interpreters agree to interpret for free at each other's family events or offer their services as pro bono for a specified number of family events per year; families use aspiring ASL interpreters based on rec-ommendations of deaf family members, certified ASL interpreters or ASL interpreter trainers; ASL interpreting agencies either reduce fees for family events or pass on the asignment, leaving the charges between the family and the recommended ASL interpreter to negotiate, with the agreement charges being lower than the agency rates; community and religious organizations supply volunteer interpreters known to the families.

Regardless of how to fund or secure ASL interpreters, without conver-sations about hiring interpreters, family harmony will *not* occur. Siblings will continue to walk on eggs with one another. "The two key elements of optimal family relationships revolve around engaging in conversations: communication among all members is clear and direct, and intimacy is prevalent and is a func-tion of frequent, equal-powered transactions" (Luterman 1987, 8–9). The more family members participating in the conversation, the better the chances for coming up with ways to share the responsibility for access. More importantly, every family member becomes part of the solution.

Just Us Two

Kay and Bree, two sisters, each told us the same Thanksgiving story occur-ring in the fictionalized story, "Just Us Two." Each graphically recalled how they were trapped, though in different ways, by isolation. Their joint efforts to confront it, with no one in the family noticing or knowing what they were doing, was their way of discreetly comforting one another so neither was alone.

This sibling pair has frequent encounters, accompanied by laughter, appreciation, respect and love for one another. Each time they run into life's inevitable conflicts, they have numerous conversations to discuss openly and honestly, work on a resolution and move on. In "Just Us Two," not only do they have the common language of ASL and deaf culture competency, and the awareness that action is necessary to forestall isolation, but as a team, they confront it with a readily available tool: the hearing sibling's willingness to *spontaneously* take on the sibling-interpreter role at a family event.

> It was Thanksgiving weekend; the sisters were at the table amidst a sea of relatives. Kay was sitting next to Grandma; Bree was across from them.
>
> KAY (catches Bree's eyes and signs at her waist): I can't stand it! Grandma's sitting inches from me and I can't talk with her! You can. Lucky you!
>
> BREE (responds rapidly): I know it's cruddy. I can't imagine how that feels. Yes ... I can. You're right. I have that privilege. I can interpret for you, if you want.
>
> Kay: No, that's not it. It is the direct contact I want with Grandma, not through someone else, even you. Grandma and I do email each other, but it's not the same like you have with her face to face or on your cell phone.
>
> BREE: I know. It sucks. And nothing has changed. (She turns her head around looking elsewhere.)
>
> KAY: What's going on?
>
> BREE: Cousin Fran is making a toast to Ivan and Dora. I'll interpret.
>
> KAY: No, please stop. You don't have to.
>
> BREE: No, I'm going to.
>
> KAY: No, you listen and relax. Period!
>
> BREE: No, I'm not leaving you out of this. Because I love you and I want you to be a part of what's going on, more than I care about the fact that I have to interpret.
>
> KAY: But I don't want you to be burdened.
>
> BREE: I'm still here. I can hear what's going on and I'm still enjoying it too. It's not painful for me to do this. Leaving you out is what hurts.

Naturally, Bree—the rescuer—jumped at the opportunity to ease the pain because she couldn't stand by as a witness. She sought the only way she knew, to use her ASL interpreting skill. The bickering between Bree and Kay, in their bubble, affirms increased tension caused by their surroundings. Do any of the relatives even notice? With no one watching, each vigorously defends their strategy for managing Kay's isolation at family gatherings. The bubble is their safety net, a place where the sisters confide in one another, and where no one else exists, because no one bothers to follow their rapid ASL.

These two adult sisters knew they wouldn't resolve their tension at family gatherings. They are always defeated by rapid chatter among hearing family members who are absorbed in their own conversations. Kay and Bree deeply yearn for the other to be a participating family member. Their argument reveals what they have to sacrifice to get there.

Being left out in the extended family is normal for Kay. As a deaf adult, she might have innumerable reasons to resist Bree's interpreting offer this time. Perhaps Kay was trying not to impose on Bree to interpret, a rule impressed on her from the time she was a child. Maybe from her years of using ASL interpreters herself, Kay is convinced Bree cannot possibly enjoy the toast like other family members, if Bree's mind and body are preoccupied with interpreting. Finally, Kay knows the emotional toll ASL interpreting takes on her sister, especially at family gatherings where Bree keeps missing opportunities to mingle with aunts, uncles and cousins. Whatever her reasons, Kay is determined to miss this toast.

Bree has had enough of deaf people being disregarded. She is adamant. It won't happen to Kay; at least not on her watch. She knew her interpreting wouldn't combat the obstacle in the room: the family that rarely took Kay into consideration. Besides, Bree sees herself as the only one who can fix the situation. Therefore she refuses to take no for an answer. All of these challenges led these sisters to formulate intimacy that gradually developed over time as they learned to depend on one another—creating trust.

In their bubble, Bree and Kay found a way to measure their monitoring success: an intimate, private place to exchange their innermost thoughts, observations, and feelings about a frequent nerve-wracking family event. The crucial element is they trust one another's judgment: Kay feels confident her sister is by her side when and if she needs her. Likewise, Bree is certain her sister will let her know when she is needed. Conversations like the one in "Just Us Two" enhanced the siblings' relationship to a deeper level, teaching these sisters to respect one another as equals, and to honor the right to have their individual needs met. Not for one second did language barriers get in the way of these siblings' quick repartee, but instead they focused on their conflict. Paramount was going beyond the pitfalls of non-signing hearing family members by negotiating the boundaries and parameters.

This vignette gives us the momentum to introduce myriad ways deaf and hearing siblings executed and fulfilled their personal commitments to one another, as individuals and as siblings. Their interactions reveal an intimacy that goes far beyond friendship, with additional rewards. Often siblings do things for one another out of their culture, traditions or family's values for lovingkindness: to care enough. Emotionally-laden acts of giving and receiving love vary in families. When siblings described their loving feelings toward their deaf family member—who is different—sometimes these feelings were beset with sympathy and pity. As one sibling, Noelle wistfully expressed, "*I don't know that he'll ever be at peace with ... what his life has been.*" Their reasoning stemmed from being eyewitnesses to the deaf member's daily challenges, so removed from their own. Ironically, deaf siblings affirmed their opposition to these very same emotions they witnessed and have been the recipients of, throughout their lives. When asked why her brother doesn't talk to her much, Audrey adamantly responded, "*Maybe he thinks deaf and hearing people are not equals.*" Yet, there were a few pairs of deaf and hearing siblings interviewed who went beyond, by empowering one another, like any committed partners would do, building on each other's strengths, and making allowances for one another's vulnerabilities.

13

Investing Quality Time

"My kid sister would wake me up to play—the first thing I saw was my hearing aid hanging in front of my eyes, close to my face."—Budd

Adult siblings have the potential to use tools or weapons that can nourish or poison their time together. Why are some relationships marked by affection and closeness and others by conflict and hostility? Sometimes what we expect from our siblings simply doesn't happen, leading to disappointment, anger or a host of other emotional responses. In addition, we make assumptions that may not be correct about why our siblings behave in ways we do not comprehend. As siblings mature, acceptance of our sibling does not mean letting go of our expectations or hope for what we want for our sibling to be. We can't change our siblings; we have the power to change ourselves. Therefore, introspection might be the first step towards improving the relationship. Refreshing our assumptions and trying to devise new ones could be more productive in creating bonds. Often deaf and hearing siblings who loved one another, believed family was important and yearned to be close, failed to break through the communication barriers. Continuing to use speech and lipreading appeared to preclude opportunities for deep, thoughtful conversations each had when they were with deaf or hearing peers.

Our role as a sibling is to feel we are valuable family members. We spend a lot of time comparing ourselves to one another, exploring diverse skills, interests and goals. In addition, we look at our feelings toward one another which affect our dignity and how we feel about ourselves. In a sense, with our siblings as our first social encounter, we continue peer training throughout our lives. As we are comparing, we are building these feelings into us being—our identity. A change-agent is paramount in the lives of Marla and her peers:

The deaf siblings I interviewed all have expressed these ideas in one way or another: We feel. We sense and know. We rightfully exist. We chose ASL because it promoted a natural connectivity, a healthy attachment to another human

160

being. Being deaf and using ASL is our self-actualization as a human being: A brain change affecting our body, mind and soul as if we are becoming a new person. These connections reveal who we truly are to the fullest as people first, and then as siblings.

Like most adults, deaf and hearing siblings are social animals, seeking companionship and friendships with each other and with people outside the family. However, we've seen that deaf and hearing siblings have a unique insidious enemy that crept into their lives, originating from a long history of ASL oppression. The result was that those siblings who did not use sign as children or adults were not only experiencing and witnessing isolation, they were also isolated from one another. At some point in their lives, deaf and hearing siblings have come to accept that hearing siblings were unable or unwilling to make learning ASL a priority. Though they were convinced in retrospect that ASL would lead them to a closer relationship, the kind they wanted, it just didn't happen. Professionals and researchers who have studied and worked with deaf people have insisted the vicious cycle of neglect in the relationship does more damage than families realize. Alan Parnes puts the ramifications of its aftereffects succinctly: "The key word is communication and without communication you have isolation. You can't have relationships without communication. If you only have minimal communication, you have minimal relationships (Parnes 2009, 9).

Sibling relationships have the potential to become a sacred friendship because of common history. Not everyone we interviewed placed a high priority on family, but those who did described themselves on the close end of Cicirelli and Gold's continuum. All used sign with one another. Those who were on the less close or hostile end of the continuum did not, but depended on lipreading and speech, with its inherent misunderstandings and guesswork, impeding natural give-and-take conversations. They paid a steep price, as Parnes describes: superficial, minimal relationships.

Is it reasonable or practical to expect your sibling to learn ASL, when it's a hearing world and hardly anyone knows ASL? Often parents have made up their minds before they had the chance to realize the consequences of their decision. These consequences have had a lasting effect on their deaf and hearing children. As adults, deaf and hearing siblings have choices. Those siblings who did not sign had regrets. Ignoring the needs of deaf siblings is similar to looking elsewhere—knowingly. Elie Wiesel once said: "The opposite of love is not hate, it's indifference. The opposite of art is not ugliness, it's indifference. The opposite of faith is not heresy, it's indifference. And the opposite of life is not death, it's indifference" (Weisel 1986, 68).

As opposed to indifference, sibling attitudes are crucial—recognizing that isolation is the enemy and becoming proactive means a commitment to combat it together. The close siblings' behavior came from the premise that deaf family members deserved to be included in family events, to make contributions to the discussion, and to be heard and seen as equally important participants with a role to play. Whatever the mechanism, it displays respect and begins to acknowledge the elephant in the room—*addressing* the exclusion of deaf family members.

14

We Will Chat Anyway

"At family gatherings, I notice they would prefer to talk with my sister, leaving me out. I wasn't mad at my sister—there was nothing I could do. I was fine with it."

—Olivia

Today's close sibling relationships resemble other friendships where frequent contacts such as email, texting, video communication, and telephone conversations as well as face-to-face interactions are used to nourish intimacy. Technology advances are sought to create opportunities for social connections: social networking sites, iPads, and other evolving accessible devices. As always with new technology, siblings may be in different places with its usage. Cell phones, for example, have taken the place of telephone booths and land-line phones in everyone's lives. However, cultural differences in how deaf and hearing people tend to approach cell phone usage may lead to tension in the relationship. For starters, deaf and hearing siblings use cell phones to stay in touch, yet their differences are in the functional use of cell phones. Since most deaf people do not use cell phones to carry on a spoken conversation, they page one another to be engaged in instant turn-taking. This may appear similar to what hearing people do to text one another, yet expectations differ surrounding the amount of information and time spent in typing messages to one another. For example, text messages by hearing people tend to be reserved for sending brief messages, rarely more than five sentences, as opposed to paged messages by deaf people used frequently to share detailed information about one's activities (Holcomb and Mindless 2009). The benefit of this technology allows deaf and hearing people to use a common language, typed English. However, typed messages may also use the syntax of ASL, which may create some confusion to those not familiar with the language.

Adult siblings, living miles from one another, are often faced with ailing parents and need to figure out how to share caretaking responsibilities. What if one sibling uses ASL and the other sibling doesn't? This is where Video Relay Service (VRS) can play a role as another technology available for bridging the communication gap. However, siblings should be aware that deaf and hearing people's tendencies using VRS may result in a potential cultural clash. "From the hearing perspective, time is a precious resource, especially in business setting" (Holcomb and Mindless 2009). This presents a challenge when VRS calls are through a third party—an ASL interpreter—where hearing people expect the calls to be brief, asking quick questions instead of engaging in lengthy discussions unless the hearing person indicates an availability to talk for longer periods.

In addition, during VRS calls, issues may arise related to moments of silence. Hearing people are generally uncomfortable with silence on their end of the call, since they are used to receiving instant feedback when talking with hearing people, using fillers like hmmm, OK, uh-huh, etc. Sometimes the silence is indicative of ASL interpreters seeing the deaf person sign and needing time to process from the visual language (ASL) to the spoken language (English). Other times, ASL interpreters neglect to notify the hearing person the deaf person left the room after the lights flashed, indicating there was someone at the door (Holcomb and Mindless 2009). In either case, the silence leaves the hearing person feeling uneasy being in the dark, with the potential for misunderstandings or hesitation to use VRS.

Adding to the complexity of VRS conversations between siblings, VRS interpreters are faced with challenges of unfamiliar family jargon: Name Signs or names to fingerspell and/or to pronounce, and/or unknown cultural and religious references. What if the family pattern allows interruptions and the VRS interpreters see this as impolite by stating, "He/she is still talking/sign-ing," thereby ignoring the family member's desire to interrupt? Turn-taking and interruptions remain at the discretion of the VRS interpreter, instead of the siblings or other parties involved who are forced to adapt.

However, more significantly, a VRS call can be a lifeline. For both deaf and hearing siblings and others, VRS conversations are functionally equivalent to spoken interactions with family members, peers, acquaintances or businesses in their lives. It is a valuable resource because an ASL interpreter is readily available 24/7 and at no cost. Unfortunately, using VRS may be perceived as the *only* tool for deaf and hearing siblings to have conversations, especially if their face-to-face encounters result in greater frustrations, disappointments, misunderstand-ings and are experienced as "failures." Lester had mixed feelings towards using interpreters, comparing face-to-face conversations with VRS interactions:

> I must say, using interpreters works great. But when I start to talk to my sister, I look at my sister, but now with an interpreter, I have to talk to the interpreter, turning my eyes away from my sister to the interpreter. But she is not my sister.

Why am I talking to her? That is why I seldom use the telephone relay system—for the same reason. I'd rather e-mail her.

Despite the potential drawbacks, VRS could be an important first step for deaf and hearing siblings to get to know one another without having to negotiate for the existence of interpreters, just to have a spontaneous live conversation in the first place! The good news with the latest technology advancement with VRS is the availability of video phones (Facetime, Skype, OoVoo, among other evolving video software programs) for deaf siblings, signing siblings and sibling-interpreters to converse in ASL. For some siblings, these software programs offer a place for lipreading as well, but they are not always the best option since video quality can be interfered with by the high-speed Internet service, resulting in increased pixels on the screen distorting the facial movements. Face-to-face video phone conversations are the ideal functional equivalence, each with video capability allowing siblings to have natural spontaneity with their common language. Yet some siblings may be so trapped in their baggage they don't take advantage of these technological and social connection opportunities to jump-start or repair relationships.

Investing in a relationship takes time involving intimacy and communication, especially with the baggage we inherit. When Mary Ann approached Judy, she addressed the goal she wanted to achieve: friendship. Mary Ann was not willing to tolerate the tension of walking on eggs with her sister. The "sit down" transformed the patterns, leading to years of intimacy between the sisters. Each was able to look at one another through a different lens and become more accepting of one another's foibles. For those siblings who want more intimate relationships by default as lifetime peers, "when working with families from a systems point of view, the emphasis is on changing patterns of interaction and not on changing individuals" (Seligman and Darling 1997, 10). "*Letting your sibling be who they are*," is what Ginger said was the crux of how she and her brother maintained a close bond with clear, healthy boundaries while addressing each other's needs. The following fictionalized story, "Changed Agent," illustrates how another pair of siblings discovered each other's best qualities and complemented the other's strengths, to combat their common enemy.

CHANGED AGENT

As the plane landed with a slight bounce, Pearl and Alex smiled at one another and breathed huge sighs of relief.

"It was a great vacation, but it's good to be back in the U.S. again," said Pearl.

"I agree! Bermuda was perfect. I loved walking on the beaches, especially the feel of the soft sand with the cool water gently massaging my feet. Most of all, I loved just spending a week with you. But I have to admit, I can't wait to sleep in my own bed and eat my own cooking."

As the plane taxied down the runway towards the terminal, the captain announced, "Please stay seated with your seat belt fastened until the plane comes to a full stop and the fasten seat belt sign goes off. It'll be just a few minutes and we'll be at the gate."

"I'd like to get off as soon as we can. My legs are feeling cramped and I need to get up, stretch and walk a bit," Alex said.

He waved at his sister to get her attention, "When we stop, I'll grab our things in the overhead bins. Are you ready? Do you have everything?"

"I have to put my book away and find my shoes under the seat."

"No problem. The plane didn't stop yet. I can tell we're still moving."

When the plane pulled into the gate and stopped, Alex felt the slight lurch forward. He also could tell that other passengers were starting to get up. He quickly unbuckled his seat belt and stood up to reach into the overhead bins. After he put on his backpack, he placed Pearl's carry-on in the aisle in front of him. "Here's yours. Got everything? Let's go!"

"Yup," Pearl replied as she stepped in front of Alex and headed down the narrow aisle towards the exit. Alex gently put his hand on Pearl's shoulder as she led the way down the meandering hallway to the immigration area. The hallway took them to a huge room, with signs showing where "U.S. Citizens" and "Non U.S. Citizens" were to line up.

Pearl stopped, looked around and said, "We need to get on the 'U.S. Citizen' line. Make sure your passport and customs papers are ready."

"Of course. Everything's ready, just like last year when we came home from Europe."

"Where's my passport?" Her right hand quivered under Alex's, while her left hand dug into her brightly colored shoulder bag.

"Keep looking!" Alex signed as he reached out to her with a reassuring pat on the shoulder.

"Look, this line is long. Dammit! There are five windows open. The other five are closed!"

"Patience. Remember the fun we had and don't fret over waiting."

"I'm trying. But it's not easy, especially because the lady behind us is gawking."

"What?"

The lady in the purple sweatsuit was mesmerized. Her eyes were glued to Pearl's moving arms and wiggling fingers. She could see Alex's hand lightly over them, following every motion. She didn't even shy away when Pearl made eye contact with her.

Pearl responded, "You know. This has happened to us before. That purple lady has been staring at us since we got off the plane. I should be used to it. I'd love to ask her, 'What's your problem? We're just having a conversation' but I won't."

Alex shrugged his shoulders, chuckling. "Relax! She's probably never seen people using Tactile Sign."

"I know. And I know I need to control myself. You're right, but it gives me the creeps and makes me mad. Anyway, people need to mind their own business."

"Well, I don't mind. Come on!" Alex signed.

"Ha. Ha. You don't mind because you don't see them staring at you!"

"Yeah, I guess that's true, but it really doesn't bother me. People are nosy and just want to know what we're doing."

"Yeah, right," Pearl snapped sarcastically. You forgive easily!"

Pearl and Alex were so engrossed, they failed to notice the line had inched forward. Pearl signed, "Pah! We're next."

A customs agent wearing a tight blue uniform brusquely came towards Pearl and Alex.

"You," he said, addressing Pearl, "can go over to booth number five,"

"And you," he continued, pointing at Alex, "can go to booth number three." As she completed her sentence, she vigorously walked away to consult with another agent for crowd control.

Pearl gasped and gripped Alex's hands, "The woman says we have to go to separate booths. Don't move. I'll explain."

Pearl started walking towards the agent. Her heart was pounding. Her palms started to sweat. As she walked away, Alex's thoughts were spinning, "This is weird. We've always been able to show our passports and papers together. Maybe things changed since 9/11.

"Gosh, didn't they notice how we're talking?"

The agent spun around and said to Pearl, "What are you doing here? Move along to the agent at booth five."

"But ... my brother is deaf and has limited vision. He needs me to interpret."

"Yeah, yeah. I've heard that before. Move on and do what I told you, otherwise we have to take you in for interrogation."

Pearl ran back to where Alex was standing. Her ASL tumbled out. "The agent thinks I'm lying. I told her I have to interpret but she says if we don't go where she told us, she will take us to a room for questioning."

Alex's face fell. "What! Questioning? Stay calm. Don't panic."

"Here she comes!" Alex felt Pearl's hands trembling and her body convulsing.

"Let me explain and you just interpret."

"I told you to move on," shouted the customs agent as she stormed up to Pearl and Alex.

As she got closer, Alex could see her outline. Alex slowly moved towards her and began to sign. Pearl took a deep breath and began speaking her brother's words. "Please listen. My sister is an ASL interpreter and she is also my guide."

"She's what? And you are ... ohhhhh. I'm so sorry. I didn't realize."

Alex placed his hand over Pearl's as she slowly signed the agent's words.

"You both can head over to booth number three. Follow me. I'll explain to the agent. Are your papers ready?" The customs agent's eyes watched Pearl's arms gracefully moving, while Alex took it all in with his hand on hers and his eyes on her face.

As adults, Pearl and Alex had what Luterman defined as "equally powered transactions." Their cumulative life experiences as a sister and brother taught each to value the other as an equal while simultaneously appropriately accommodating each other's needs. Pearl clearly enunciated all the facets of an exemplary sibling relationship: "*Your brothers and your sisters—they're all no different than you are. We all have our own needs. You know, we all want to be included. We all want to be accepted."* Seeing is believing. Proactively, this brother and sister put their heads together, negotiated and took action to overcome a common obstacle in their lives—the hearing world's ignorance of the deaf-blind person's needs. Their collaborative efforts contrast sharply with another sibling pair who were raised in a different era: Nathan and Simon.

Nathan and Simon's family was unique—they grew up in a deaf household. Their parents' friends, leading members of the close-knit deaf community, were frequent visitors in their home. Like many deaf families of the time, the brothers' family absorbed the hostility that permeated society: being deaf was a stigma, spoken English was a necessity for getting along in the hearing world, and ASL was an inferior gesture system, not to be equated with English. In his interview Simon said he grew up in a time when *"deaf people were viewed by a lot of normal people as abnormal."* Being the only hearing member in the house, he naturally gravitated to someone whom he perceived as normal. The family housekeeper of Irish ancestry became his childhood confidante. Her hearing status and her spoken English made her more equal or more like him than his own flesh and blood.

During their interviews, both brothers acknowledged that despite satisfactory oral communication between them, they wished they were closer. Simon and Nathan rarely see one another except at family life-cycle events, in contrast to Pearl and Alex, who take frequent vacations together. Simon equated his hearing status with being normal. Therefore, his brothers, as well as his parents, were not given a chance to have "equal-powered transactions" with him. To illustrate the damaging effects of stigma attached to being deaf, Nathan described a frequent occurrence when Simon would rush them across the street to avoid deaf people signing. Each time it happened, he felt personally humiliated. The lingering shame of being an integral part of a signing family precluded a relationship with Simon. This is in sharp opposition to Pearl and Alex, who comfortably used Tactile Sign in public in spite of people staring, and loved being seen together.

Echoing Pearl's words: *"Letting our siblings be who they are"* inscribes them as partners, granting acknowledgment of their unique differences. Mutual respect and acceptance of one another are two critical items missing in Nathan and Simon's relationship. In Nathan's eyes, Simon's avoidance behavior was a rejection of deaf people, their language and a community Nathan cherished. As history has shown, during Simon and Nathan's formative years, the term *deaf* was a stigmatized label. The term included stereotypes ingrained in society's view of deaf people: they were deaf and dumb imbeciles, looked down upon, and in general denigrated. However, in Pearl and Alex's family the labels *deaf* or *deaf-blind* were seen as attributes identifying Alex within the deaf community, with no negative connotations. Additionally, since both siblings have readily accepted one another's cultures where communication involving sound and touch are drastically different, Pearl's role in the deaf community, as a hearing sibling and as an ASL interpreter working with deaf and deaf-blind individuals, affirms that using their tactile communication is just another way to talk. Jelica Niccio and A.J. Granda, two deaf-blind activists of an evolving movement called Pro-Tactile, are promoting additional cultural strategies to enhance tactile communication. Their techniques are primarily about touching, which could be gentle knee-tapping or tapping on the forearm, which function as the equivalent of facial expressions used by sighted signer, to acknowledge they are still engaged in the conversation. Sibling who use these techniques are treating one another as equal participants, improving the natural give-and-take in their conversations.

Why were Nathan and Simon unable to relinquish the pervasive beliefs that had permeated their lives? Perhaps the scars in their psyches ran too deep. Was the stigma so profound in this deaf family they couldn't take advantage of the tool they knew existed? Fast-forward fifty years, when ASL has become the norm in many *deaf* families with deaf and hearing children. None could fathom being without it where learning by osmosis is an everyday event through accessible shared language.

Conversations Lead the Way to Intimacy

The stories of the twenty-two siblings we met give hope for those who yearn for a change. Their examples show us how some moved on to the next level of intimacy. Those who found the courage to confront and risk change believed there was enough common ground to have a sibling in their lives. Nadia's incentive to learn sign was to join her siblings as a threesome. She gained a brother, instead of a deaf sibling, and a tighter relationship with her sister. Micki tried to bring Enid into her DEAF-WORLD, but both sisters admitted their attempt for intimacy was inhibited by their language differences. In contrast, although Terrence and Haley grew up with a common language and are extremely close, Terrence's laid-back and Haley's hung-strung personality differences may either interfere with or nurture their interactions from moving onto the next intimate level.

Healthy families don't sweep conflicts under the rug where they continue corroding family relations. Instead, they "address conflicts as they arise" (Luterman and Ross 1991, 59). However, how can families, including several we interviewed, get beyond the deaf attribution? Blaming the fact of being deaf or ignoring inappropriate behavior does not resolve conflicts between deaf and hearing siblings. Building sibling relationships starts in the early years.

When parents tell their children: "Let it go. He's deaf," they are condoning inappropriate behavior and unintentionally encouraging resentment between siblings. Justification is used as a neutralizer to settle conflicts, but its effectiveness is short-lived because it buries the issue deeper. If a deaf child hits his hearing sister, it's easy to say, "He didn't understand you. He's deaf. Let it go," instead of addressing both behaviors. "Your brother hit you because he misunderstood what you said," needs to be accompanied by, "Hitting is not acceptable behavior," then followed up with whatever the family does to discipline and provide positive reinforcement for good behavior. However, this intervention requires parents and siblings to be sufficiently fluent in ASL to understand one another, a feature lacking in many families.

There continues to be a great deal of finger-pointing in families where it is easy to shift the conflicts to the deaf card. For example, "He is angry because we didn't learn ASL growing up," or "These two are hearing, therefore they are not close with me because I am deaf," or "She got away with this because she is deaf!" Parents and hearing siblings are not the only ones who blame deaf issues as the cause of conflict. Some deaf siblings may internalize misunderstanding and blame a negative event on being deaf. At times, situations arise where deaf people are in a hearing environment and everything seems to revolve around their being deaf, not allowing other facets of their identities to appear or flourish that might ameliorate the situation. Similar experiences may occur with religious people who maintain that identity while coexisting in society that has different beliefs. If healthy families address the deaf attribution early on together as a unit, rather than letting it fester, and identify nourishing tools that feed everyday interactions, they would alleviate the burden of daily communication and isolation challenges.

Using Cicirelli and Gold's continuum is a starting place for siblings to begin identifying themselves on the continuum and where they would like their relationship to be. However, as a deciding factor to the intensity of closeness, several sibling pairs defined their close relationships based on meaningful, as opposed to superficial, conversations. Sign and/or ASL, their common childhood language, was *the* critical tool making conversations possible in the first place, to even have a relationship. Therefore, their meaningful conversations became the gateway to opportunities for investing the time to achieve a greater level of depth in the relationship. As a team, the sibling pairs not only encouraged their relatives to learn ASL but their model of signing to one another provided an incentive to be part of conversations involving the deaf family member.

Sharing one another's culture is an additional treasure—often the subject of meaningful conversations about an event: a play, a finals match in tennis or a museum tour. The DEAF-WORLD is not culturally limited. It is abundant with deaf theater, deaf arts, ASL animations, ASL poetry, deaf humor, international Deaflympics and many more. Signing siblings and sibling-interpreters' lives have been enriched and rewarded by their involvement in the deaf community, including advocacy, ASL and ASL interpreting politics. Each time deaf and hearing sibling pairs spend time together, deaf siblings gain insights to the hearing world, and are introduced to the positive features of a world many are led to believe is against them.

Eavesdropping is an addictive tool whereby signing siblings and sibling-interpreters keep deaf siblings apprised of surrounding sounds affecting the tone of sound-oriented events: plates crashing, an aunt bursting out laughing or a grandfather's storytelling of his childhood days in Europe. Access entices meaningful conversations, entailing more information-sharing and a willingness to pick up more ASL, all of which foster siblings to be attuned to one another's personalities, interests, and quirks. For some siblings who are attuned and sensitive to the severity of the isolation, monitoring—achieved by eavesdropping—often leads to rescuing communication breakdowns based on subtle or direct signals from deaf siblings.

Personal relationships are built based on intimate conversations in social settings compared to formal settings. Chitchat, seemingly about nothing, may not seem important to interpret and be bothered with, but it is often the foundation of relationship-building. What dress you wear to the interview, what candidate you send money to, tells all about who you are and what you believe in. When family members push one another's buttons in ways that dismiss the deaf sibling, signing siblings and sibling-interpreters' blood boils because they've lived the benefits of chit-chat towards getting to know family members. By depriving deaf siblings access to conversations where they miss the information hearing people learn by osmosis, deaf family members are at a huge disadvantage, or worse, they get misconstrued and labeled as incapable or socially awkward. Do we create an unfair playing field based on lack of sound-access? Why don't we acknowledge this reality: if deaf siblings didn't *see* something happen, they weren't party to it. Hearing siblings who keep their deaf siblings in the loop have respect for their deaf sibling as an equal who has the right to as much sound information as they, to know about the hearing world around them.

Several siblings had conversations about the drawbacks surrounding hiring ASL interpreters for family events, relatives and friends who do not sign. While it may have been intended as a strategy to break the isolation cycle, deaf and hearing siblings both acknowledged it's a temporary fix. Sporadic use of ASL interpreters never made up for lost years of chit-chat and relationship-building conversations with one another or relatives. However, hiring ASL interpreters *is* a practical tool with no guarantees: meaningful conversations are dependent on individuals' personalities, interests and whether they have a desire to get to know the sibling or relatives.

Attitude Counts

Siblings who claim they were best friends instantly knew attitude was the key. They also understood how the history of oppression colored both deaf and hearing siblings' world views toward people who are different. As a response, signing siblings and sibling-interpreters proactively took action, making it very personal, tackling the vicious cycle of patronization and stigma, and recognizing that oppressors may be in their backyard—colleagues, educators, parents or relatives. For Judy, meeting and sharing stories with other siblings felt like a validation.

> The signers I interviewed, like the younger me of many years ago, knew enough to pick up new vocabulary and kept on interpreting to ensure their deaf siblings' participation. It was enormously satisfying to know I wasn't the only one. I was also filled with envy at those siblings who had grown up signing and had respect for deaf culture and understood the oppression. They grew up consciously knowing and doing something about it rather than feeling the helplessness I experienced as a child.

Growing up with a sibling who is seen as defective, or who sees himself as defective, precludes "equally powered transactions." Meaningful conversations only occur between people who see themselves as siblings first, and hearing status as just another attribute, like physical appearances, personalities, or talents. Echoing Dr. Martin Luther King's dream: siblings should not be judged by their hearing status, but by their character. In reality, as Marla demonstrates, many families never get beyond the disability label.

> For a while I believed I was "special," which kept me at a distance. It was quite an ego booster until I realized the attribution special had a different meaning, Being treated special became a constant reminder I was different and that being different must have meant the deaf attribution. Is this something my parents, siblings, and other people, including me, should get beyond? How about the chance to see me for who I am, not what I achieve?

The deaf attribution may have positioned Marla to work harder to overcome whatever came her way. It may be her reality, yet "One is not privileged based on being seen as 'special' or what one has accomplished. Privilege is not about being seen as an individual but as being seen as part of a social category" (Tuccoli 2008, 7–8). As social beings, people relate to one another as "insiders" and "outsiders," responding to whether they share the same values and interests, or have the chemistry to connect. "She has the right attitude" is a common phrase describing a person who does not share the attributes of being different, but affirms that person as an ally. In the case of deaf attribution, the attitude begins with the first step—to embrace the difference. Marla's brother, Joseph, advises parents and siblings to "*be sensitive to the deaf culture. Not as a handicap to fix, rather as a unique culture that has its own special aspects or sensitivities.*" In retrospect, it is a process of recognition and acceptance of the person, not the disability. But he added, "*It takes age and maturity to understand that.*" For some siblings, this may be applicable just as it is with other aspects of their lives. Yet, many siblings were taught at a very early age their sibling is just like them.

Some people who sign say they didn't know there was a hearing world until they entered the DEAF-WORLD. By default, deaf and hearing siblings coexist in either world. However, some siblings we interviewed are "out of touch" with the DEAF-WORLD and are largely unaware that the privileges they are using might offend their deaf siblings. Any time a conversation occurs, hearing siblings have a choice whether they want to tune out any environmental sounds interfering with their ability to carry on a conversation with a deaf family member. Often, turning their heads towards the external sound makes it difficult for siblings to validate and respect the eye-contact necessary for conversations with a deaf sibling. Conversations with a deaf person require cultural feedback like nodding, a quizzical look, or other facial expression similar to the "uh huh," "hmmm" in spoken conversations—all of which affirm positive engagement. Validation and having respect for one's thoughts and feelings give siblings ample opportunities to understand one another intimately. When siblings have conversations about "It sucks the way these hearing cousins act awkwardly each time they see me" or "I'd love to stay and chat but my kids have school tomorrow and we need to leave," it shows they are in this together, not alone. Often reality interferes and they can't always resolve access or other issues that arise. One way to alleviate the burden is to get family members to address these issues responsibly and constantly support one another: to be aware, stay alert, discuss and agree on ways for siblings to combat the inevitable isolation for the rest of their lives. When all else fails, humor is an excellent stress-buster.

Suppose deaf and hearing siblings were to recognize that deaf people have many gifts edifying humanity? They might learn about the enormous contributions deaf people have made to literature, art, poetry, sports, language, science, technology, linguistics, education, psychology, medicine and sociology. Even if people are aware a DEAF-WORLD exists, most know little about it. Some may have noticed deaf people signing in a restaurant, encountered a deaf person at work, sat next to a deaf student in a class, or perhaps only seen deaf people from afar, on television or in the movies. The average John Q. Public, if he's had any firsthand experience, recognizes deaf people as different, having no connection or little impact on their lives. Yet most have probably believed the unspoken message, like some of the siblings we met, that being deaf is a tragedy and not a desirable quality or trait to live by. Some siblings might be unaware of the origins of their deeply rooted belief they acquired from the medical establishment that curing deaf people should not be questioned. Then there are siblings who totally see being deaf is only small part of who the deaf person is. It is how, *as siblings*, they react to the circumstances surrounding the deaf issue that carries deaf and hearing siblings throughout their lives in positive and healthy ways.

By the time the siblings we interviewed read this book, many may have changed their feelings about their siblings. We recognize change is naturally evolving as people adapt their identities within their families, are influenced by their jobs, social circles and other outside or internal stimuli. If we go back to biblical times, we will see deaf people represented a part of humanity that were employed and earned respect: "You shall not curse the deaf; you shall not put a stumbling block before the blind, but you shall fear your God" (Leviticus 19:23). Even though there may be numerous interpretations to the biblical translations, we need to recognize that "they" are just like us. Therefore, it all becomes relative to embrace what it means to be human. Defining humanity can be seen by some deaf and hearing siblings as a feature of cognitive dissonance: holding the belief that being deaf is both a positive and a negative condition. The arguments surrounding the beliefs depend on one's perception, but in reality it is the society-ingrained view that creates the attribution and stigma of *disability*. Though attitudes may be deeply held within the family, adults have the capacity to change, for all to benefit.

A new interest in the mainstream society has been taking place. Ironically, growing in numbers exponentially, hearing parents are seeking baby ASL books, DVDs, or other media forms to learn signs with hearing infants, stimulating ASL vocabulary at an earlier age. On the other hand, parents with deaf children are pulled in different directions regarding language acquisition and advised to use: ASL, all forms of MCE systems, Cued Speech, use amplification of various kinds, or to speak only.

Cities where large deaf populations reside have high schools and colleges offering ASL classes; often a small percentage is taught by deaf professionals. As a result of ASL's being placed on the list in the Modern Language Association's *MLA International Bibliography* as a "natural" language back in 1998, the Association of Departments of Foreign Language's (ADFL) 2002 survey showed that "among undergraduates and graduates at four-year (or plus) colleges, ASL ranked fifth in language course enrollments, with Spanish, French, German and Italian placing ahead of it" (Brueggemann 2009, 31). Often opportunities arise for the two worlds to be drawn together by their common language, ASL. Students meet and mingle with other signers, to increase their ASL fluency, as a requirement for these classes or at cultural events hosted by ASL programs on campus or off-campus, or possibly in partnerships with local deaf community organizations. Additionally, the enforcement of the ADA as a civil rights law as well as the IDEA school laws have opened the gates to even more interactive opportunities for deaf and hearing people. Employers, medical establishments, recreational and public facilities as well as government agencies are accountable: provide access, address equal participation, and most importantly, enforce the law challenging existing behavior of exclusion, isolation and indifference.

To break the vicious cycle of neglect, something on a more personal level beyond enforcing existing laws needs to happen. As deaf people look for work, they often encounter people who have taken one or two ASL courses, who express regret that they haven't maintained their signing skills. The workplace is a venue where administrators have the potential to hire deaf people who use ASL, to encourage their companies to work side by side with them, thereby increasing the opportunities for employees to use ASL. In addition, everyone can benefit from visual interactions such as using eye contact, interpreting body language or other cultural aspects of ASL.

At the same time, despite the widespread availability of ASL classes, many state and privately funded deaf schools are closing. Throughout the country deaf children remain isolated in mainstreamed classes with few or no deaf peers and rare exposure to deaf adults, restricting their immersion in the larger deaf community where they would benefit from the experiences of deaf role models.

Despite the excitement taking place by those new to the DEAF-WORLD and the enthusiasm of ASL students, when a family receives the diagnosis their child is deaf, the stigma reappears and the Milan Impact persists. Families, siblings included, with help from medical providers and other policy makers, begin the long road to deal with the tragic event, constantly searching for a fix or a cure. It begins with parents being told of a *failed* hearing test at the hospital a few hours after birth. Suppose medical professional react differently at the very start of the family's journey? What needs to be done to cease the vicious cycle that has endured for more than 125 years? How crucial is it for families, specifically siblings, to get beyond the stigma and begin to have conversations about ways to pursue positive and nurturing relationships?

Families with deaf members constitute a rare occurrence, since in the United States "there are approximately 200,000 people who were either born deaf or lost their hearing before they acquired spoken language, and who use sign language as their primary form of communication" (Marschark 1997, 24). With so few role models for families to learn from, deaf and hearing siblings expend a great deal of energy just figuring out how to interact with one another. Not one of the siblings we interviewed had ever participated in adult-led discussions about having a deaf or hearing sister or brother where they might have learned more about the value of acceptance of one another in the way that Eckhart Tolle, an internationally recognized spiritual teacher, defines *acceptance*: "Performing an action in the state of acceptance means you are at peace while you do it. Acceptance means: For now, this is what this situation, this moment, requires me to do, and so I do it willingly" (Tolle 2005, 296).

Only if we learn from deaf and hearing siblings who are involved in each other's lives, will we know what may benefit us. As authors we readily admit our interview with deaf and hearing siblings gave us mere "snapshots" of significant events in their lives, stories they chose to share with us. Our focus was to provide an inside look into the interactions between adult deaf and hearing siblings and an analysis on how well they know one another. As we've noted in our pilot study using Cicirelli and Gold's continuum of relationships, based on the siblings' interactions with one another, some siblings have clearly invested in one another's lives, while others did so sporadically, rarely or never. Some were boiling with anger or resentment and unable to move on, others were attempting to make amends with their sisters and brothers, while others considered themselves to be best friends. The common threads are that the siblings were all striving to find their place in the family. Some were stuck in defined roles from their childhoods, others changed over time, moving into new roles that were more satisfying or at least less stressful. Most remarkable yet not surprising is that the siblings, as adults, are still evolving, strategizing to locate the boundaries of their comfort zones while interacting with their sibling.

Two thumbprints were evident permeating the most satisfying relationships between deaf and hearing siblings: realization that the deaf attribution was no longer visible, and that ASL no longer belonged *only* to deaf people. Being siblings is what they were to one another. Their identities no longer are labeled as deaf or hearing, nor did they disregard their distinctive cultural mannerisms. Crucial to their bonding was the natural "give-and-take" interactions through use of their common language, ASL. A necessary venture for sharing experiences was their immersion in the DEAF-WORLD. These deaf and hearing siblings were "active listeners," observing the mannerisms critically used by ASL users. For example, a sign of being attentive during conversations with three or more people is turn-taking in a circle facing one another, rather than people talking at the same time within proximity or at a distance. Maintaining eye contact is another visual cue showing respect for the person talking. These siblings also strived, though not always successfully, to involve as many family members as possible in the decision-making process surrounding access to communication, recognizing everyone deserves an equal chance to participate at family events. Interpersonal relationships can flourish each time siblings and their families talk openly and honestly about the elephant in the room—the relentless isolation of deaf siblings—and everyone shares the responsibility for communication issues. Commitment and follow-through by learning ASL, recognizing the positive attributes of being deaf contributing to the family's well-being, and sharing the responsibility for hiring and paying for ASL interpreters when needed, eventually leads families a step closer to harmony.

Deaf and hearing siblings enjoying each other, seeking common interests, and engaging in discussions of their most intimate thoughts have lifelong confidants, playmates, and friends: a triple blessing. Siblings like Kay and Bree; Alex, Pearl and Nadia; and Judy and Larry, all are evidence that when they embrace one another as equals, their role as allies become cemented in each other's lives. And they entrusted us with reasons to celebrate:

> *"Letting your brothers and sisters be who they are and have them be your brother or sister first."*
> —Pearl, hearing sibling

> *"She's my sister. That we are deaf and hearing was never an issue."*
> —Kay, deaf sibling

MOVING ON

Siblings! Are we ready to tackle the hard conversations we've avoided?
If we act, we may find the outcome is better than we ever dreamed possible
Because—it's about us, not about our sibling. What will we to do to have an ally?
Let others help us to jump-start conversations: therapist, mediator, a trusted friend.
It may be emotional, even painstaking, but
No pain, no gain. so
Gather ideas from others who've walked in our shoes—like a sibshop or any support group.
Can we create our own framing with fresh perspectives?
One sibling's memory of an event is as valid as another's.
Not right or wrong. It's yours, mine and our story. Period.
Vow to move on, search for common ground with activities to enjoy.
Every step leads the way to safe places where stimulating opportunities for chats occur.
Realize our sibling's priorities may not be ours but theirs to own, not for us to judge.
Sisters and brothers may have different expectations about what they want.
Attitudes, feelings and actions don't change overnight but can with
Time.
If we give it our best, then we know we've tried.
Or—one of us can make that first move—deciding that it's worth the gamble.
No one can anticipate how our sister or brother will respond to us reaching out.
Surely, if we don't, the status quo will remain. Will it work for us?

Appendix A:
Continuum of Intensities
of Sibling Closeness

A Continuum of Intensities of Sibling Closeness is an opportunity for siblings to engage in conversations to identify and explore the degree of closeness they have with their siblings.

A CONTINUUM OF INTENSITIES
OF SIBLING CLOSENESS

Where are you with your sibling?

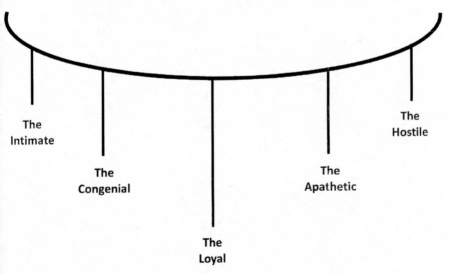

The
Intimate

The
Congenial

The
Loyal

The
Apathetic

The
Hostile

Where are you with your sibling?

Definitions of Intensities of Sibling Closeness

- **The Intimate**—adult siblings are especially close and extremely devoted. They value their relationship above all others.
- **The Congenial**—adult siblings are friends. They are close and caring but place a higher value on their marriage and parent-child relationships.
- **The Loyal**—adult siblings base their relationship on their common family history. They maintain regular, periodic contact, participate in family gatherings, and support each other during times of crisis.
- **The Apathetic**—adult siblings feel indifferent toward each other. They rarely are in contact.
- **The Hostile**—adult siblings are based on anger, resentment, and very negative feelings.

Appendix B:
Questions for
Guided Discussion

1. What was unique about the book? Identify specific themes the authors discussed throughout the book.
2. In what way has the information the authors presented been interesting and/or insightful, made you uncomfortable or prompted you to change your perspective?
3. Consider historical and cultural events that are similar or different from the Milan Effect.
4 Describe the possible benefits of using ASL in your life.
5. Identify examples of being stigmatized in your life. How has it affected you?
6. Describe the roles you play in your family compared to the roles described in the book: monitor, facilitator, protector, etc. Consider not only your role as a sibling but the other roles you take on as well: daughter, son, uncle, cousin, grandparent, etc.
7. Using your own experience, what do you consider nurtures or inhibits the closeness of siblings?
8. If you knew you had a few months to live, what would you want to tell your sibling(s)?
9. How do the parents' decisions regarding language acquisition, educational placement and social development shape the bonds between deaf and hearing siblings? What are the consequences, as it relates to siblings, if parents decide not to learn ASL?
10. Consider the forces that contribute to the rebellion of deaf or hearing siblings when they want their family members to use ASL. Discuss

the changing nature of the relationship among the deaf and hearing siblings who didn't sign as children but did as adults.

11. In the stories presented in the book, discuss examples of Audism.

12. "She is my sister. That we are deaf or hearing was never an issue." Discuss the semantics of this quote and provide possible ways to live by this. Compare and contrast the perspectives of disability with that of minority culture and how these views may have affected the person's quote.

Appendix C:
Let's See What
Our Fingers Know

We've been asked quite often: how did two people, living three states apart, write a book together? In spite of having taken many years to complete this work, the process could not be done autonomously. Many colleagues of ours had co-authored books, often writing different chapters independently and then editing one another's work. While that recipe worked for them, their strategy felt unnatural to us. We needed to interact with one another, have face-to-face time to blend our ideas, each phrase and every word.

Back in 2002, we didn't have the tools for interactive conversations. In the meantime, sending one another drafts through emails was a step closer to working together, yet these emails held us back. Although technology such as TTY and text relay service was available, we rejected them. TTYs entailed that we take turns typing and end our chunks of our suggestions for sibling themes with Go Ahead (GA), permitting the other person to begin typing, or Stop Keying (SK) to end the conversation. Text relay service involved a communication assistant (CA) as the third party between a TTY user and a landline phone user.

In 2005, we attempted to use the latest technology, America Online (AOL) AIM-Chat, but it was cumbersome and barely could be called interactive! Each of us would type a topic into a box associated with our screen name while looking at and cutting and pasting it into our proposed manuscript, a separate document on our computers. The challenge was the AOL AIM-Chat conversation was in a vertical heap, stressing our eyeballs as we hunted for where we left off. In the very same year, software programs such as Skype, OoVoo and others in conjunction with high-speed Internet were emerging, yet they were unintelligible for ASL conversations, transforming us into mechanized robots with ghosts shadowing every move of our hands, body language, and facial expressions.

Suddenly, video relay service companies serving the deaf community created videophones (VP) that made our face-to-face conversations in ASL possible. A videophone "is a telephone with a video display, capable of simultaneous video and audio for communication between people in real-time." VPs use advanced technology video software programs in conjunction with high-speed Internet and webcams on any hardware device (laptops, handhelds) or TV monitors to allow users to see one another. To expedite our work on the manuscript we used Google's technology feature, Google documents (G-doc). The duality of using VP and G-doc technology was the magical ingredient that put us in the same room, on the same page at the same time, like being on the phone together. Sounds simple? Not quite. Picture us:

> So if I'm watching Marla either signing or fingerspelling about something we just wrote or something she wants me to look at, I can't look at our manuscript on my computer screen while she's using ASL because she's on my TV screen, three feet adjacent at a different angle. Ditto in reverse. Any time we break eye contact to look at or add something to our manuscript, our conversation is cut off. Our peripheral vision occasionally catches a hand wave, if we dare to interrupt one another to stop typing.

So if we do not look at our manuscript on G-docs and the VP simultaneously, how do we identify what the other is talking about?

> JUDY: Do you see my purple paragraph?
> MARLA: [Shaking head.]
> JUDY: Look under the blue one.
> MARLA: Can we merge the two? These two are the ideas we want. The rest is repetitive.
> JUDY: I'll copy and paste it. You write above it and I'll write below. OK?

Using colors to identify was quicker than Signing every word.

We also found our totally different writing styles complemented one another, which led us to balance our perspectives. Judy's tendencies are detailed-oriented: "*I* would just dump all my random thoughts on the page in paragraph form as my goal was to get them down on paper." Whereas Marla's approach was quite the contrary, envisioning the overall organization of the text: "I have the main ideas and the sequence in my head. Using bullets and expanding these ideas into an outline, I created a flow chart. Someone had to keep track of where we were and where we were going—I guess that was me who took on the huge task!"

One more bonus neither of us anticipated. Through our ASL conversations and writing together in English, we each had the opportunity to fine-tune our second language skills. And our conversations became the "driver" for the development of the text:

MARLA: Why don't we create a variety of genres—fictionalized stories, highlighted quotes from our interviews, and our journals in our text?

JUDY: Yes! I should've known—you've always been the drama queen!

MARLA: And ... you're the comma drama! I see it all over your first drafts—seasoned with commas everywhere.

JUDY: [Looking at the draft] I know, but you've got the knack for dissecting key words, catching every nuance of meaning ... your edits on my dull text are awesome! Did Bree really put it that way or did we put words in her mouth?

MARLA: Can you go back to the original interview and double check? Use that fabulous search engine—Agent Ransack—that Peter got for you. By the way, this highlighted sentence seems clear to me, yet I see your face is not quite satisfied. What's the matter?

JUDY: I'm not sure. Let me see if my fingers know.

MARLA: Pah! You nailed it!

JUDY: I know. But I didn't think it in my head. How'd it come out my fingers, onto the keyboard and on the screen?

MARLA: LOL. Don't ask me. I'm clueless but the creative process is a fun mystery. By the way, I see two purple sentences below and they don't work for me.

JUDY: Which parts didn't you like? I agree the second sentence needs reworking but what's wrong with the first?

MARLA: Everyone's written about that and said that. Dig deeper.

JUDY: Fair enough, but this is just plain hard! I don't think it's related to us working in two languages. Agree?

MARLA: Yes! The content is a challenge. To say what we want to say as well as to stay faithful to the stories siblings shared with us.

JUDY: I guess that's why the revisions of those two purple sentences just cost us an hour and a half!

Colleagues, friends and family once again often asked us why it took us three hours to barely cover a page. People assumed the two languages, English and ASL, might have been the reason it took us so long to write the book. Wrong. Being bilingual and bicultural made it easier—we had an abundance of both languages and cultural competencies literally and figuratively in our hands.

Our different approaches to expressing ourselves remained a challenge, requiring us to take time to understand one another's ideas or even get ideas across, cautiously broaching topics that might push the other's buttons. Yet we moved on once we had the meta-conversation about it.

MARLA: We're missing the nuance. The English revision lost the flavor of the ASL. Maybe either you do not understand my point or I wasn't making myself clear. Let me rephrase though it feels like I've said it several times already.

JUDY: Try me again. We have to keep going. Did you mean ... ?

MARLA: Sort of ... but do you think we could move the first sentence to the end and then put the blue one in the purple paragraph? The flow works better.

JUDY: Show me. You hold it in your head. I have to see it.

MARLA: OK. Let me move it around. We'll keep the original so you can compare the difference.

JUDY: Ooops! Google kicked me off.

MARLA: Yeah, your red viewer icon is gone! LOL.

JUDY: have no patience for this. Dammit! Without our conversations, we can't move on!

MARLA: Amen!

Appendix D:
BMJ Family
Interpreter Fund
by Judith A. Jonas

For years my brother, sister and I had been sharing the costs of interpreters for family gatherings. Our family email list—called BMJ for Brick Mendelson Jonas—that keeps all of us in touch with one click, are our children and their families, and some cousins. We used the email list to reach out to the next generation with the focus to ensure a *continuation of interpreter presence at family gatherings,* after our generation passes on.

One summer in 2008, one of my nephews asked me and my brother for advice about hiring interpreters for his daughter's Bat Mitzvah. His query led the family to a discussion on the topic of hiring interpreters not only for that event, but for future gatherings as well. Daniel and his wife belong to a congregation in Rochester, New York, a city with a fairly large concentration of deaf people attending the National Technical Institute for the Deaf at Rochester Institute of Technology (RIT), and the Rochester School for the Deaf. Their temple was used to hiring and paying for interpreters for their religious services. In the process of arranging interpreters for Megan's Bat Mitzvah, they asked Daniel about having the interpreter stay for the reception following the ritual. Unsure of the details with the hiring process, Daniel then asked my brother and me: *"Can you guys advise?*

After many discussions among me and my husband, my brother, our nephew and our children about the complexities that come with hiring interpreters at our family events, Larry broadened the topic in an email to me, leading with his concerns about the future:

I appreciate the suggestion to bring it up with the whole BMJ Family. Out of concern for Kelby and Karina having access when Carolyn and I pass on, I was thinking of putting aside funds from my estate specifically to cover interpreter costs as long as there is a deaf family member. Then I started wondering why I should take responsibility for this. I think one of many possible ways to handle this would be to set up a fund with annual dues from each household where the oldest member of the household is above the age of 25 and working full time (i.e., not still in school). If something along these plans are acceptable, then we'd need a volunteer to oversee the fund and take care of the costs. I would suggest that it be one of the third generation group. How's this for starters to get the discussion going to generate different ideas and input?

Further consensus was building among the older generation to draw in more family members for input on this issue. The following email went out to the BMJ family:

To: The BMJ Family—the next generation
From: Uncle Larry, Aunt Carolyn, Aunt Judy, Uncle Peter and Uncle Gene
Re: BMJ Family Interpreter Fund: A proposal
Date: 7/24/2009

Most of you are aware that we of the older generation have been funding interpreter services for family events for decades. We plan to continue to contribute. However, since we are aging, we feel it's appropriate to ask the next generation to assume some responsibility. Most of us agree that the presence of paid interpreters has made it possible for all of us to enjoy easy communication with one another, without "burdening" those family members who sign.

We propose that the informal "BMJ Family Interpreter Fund" move into the hands of the younger generation. So we ask:

—that members of the next generation join us in contributing to this ongoing BMJ Family Interpreter Fund, and
—that an individual from that next generation volunteer, perhaps on a rotating basis, to take on the fund's management.

Our generation will start the BMJ Family Interpreter Fund at $300 and suggest that this be the targeted minimum. This figure is based on past interpreter costs at various affairs such at Bar/Bat Mitzvahs, Passovers, etc. As an example, below are interpreter costs of the last 4 family events:

4/23/08	$ 140	Passover
7/19/08	$ 175	Mary-Ann's funeral
4/4/09	$ 280	Jacob's Bar Mitzvah
4/8/09	$ 180	Passover

We suggest the job of the volunteer would be:

—Keep track of the fund, pay interpreter bills, and receive contributions.
—Every time the fund goes below $300, send an email requesting contributions to build up the fund.
—Let everyone know annually how much is on hand, the total amount col-

lected during the year (not individual contributions!), and each specific expenditure.

The above proposal is open for discussion with the goal of reaching a consensus. The next event is Megan's Bat Mitzvah. Daniel and Linda's temple has offered to cover the interpreter costs during the Bat Mitzvah services but we need to cover the costs of interpreters for the reception. Personally, we plan to fund that portion, ideally via the new BMJ Family Interpreter Fund, in the spirit of unity.

Any volunteers? Once a volunteer is located, we'll send our checks to that person.

What follows are some of the family members' thoughts, edited for brevity:

- Daniel, our nephew, one of the first who responded: Honestly, make it far less complicated. Just say you are starting a fund and that everyone who wishes to support it should send a few dollars your way.... It is not a matter of taking "responsibility" so much as a matter of you voting with your dollars for what you believe in.
- Mona, Daniel's sister, chimed in: I second both of Daniels remarks—a) Put out a request and let people send what they will. b) It is a nice legacy you can leave to the family. There will be a constant reminder every time it is used.
- Wendy, Judy's daughter: I like Daniel's idea—just ask people to contribute. Someone should be "in charge" of collecting money/keeping an account. Whenever that account runs low, send another e-mail requesting $$. The person "in charge" should rotate every couple of years too.
- Kelby, Larry's youngest son: I concur with Daniel. I think the estate idea is a great way to go if that's something you're interested in.
- Deborah, Judy's daughter: We will happily contribute, and prefer that the fund coordinator recommend a per family contribution amount (recognizing that some families will still give a bit more and some less depending on financial circumstances at the time).
- Steve and Carmen (Judy and Larry's nephew and his wife): I agree with Deborah. Steve thinks it's probably easier to just set up some kind of family annual dues ... depending on how many families we are talking about, could be about $25 per family per year, and as Deb said, those that are willing to send in a bit more, can. Overall we think it's a great idea and agree that it's time to pass the torch to the next generation.

As the consensus was building, behind-the-scenes discussion continued amongst the older generation and humor made its way, through our brother-in-law, into the serious discussion about finding a "volunteer" to coordinate the fund:

To All:
Regarding the above: WE HAVE A VOLUNTEER! Wendy!! (After threatening to bite her on her big toe. Chris said I could).

Her Job Description:

1. Set up a list of members by family.
2. Ask you to send her an opening contribution of $30 per family. (You can start sending her money now.)
3. Discuss with her Uncle Larry to determine what interpreting services would be needed for what events.
4. Talk to her mother to decide the best way to contact and set up the times an interpreter is needed.
5. Train her replacement (No, it can't be Evan [her son, who was 6 at the time]).
6. Get thanked by a grateful Family.
7. Run a contest (the winner goes to Paris, France for the weekend) to come up with a name for this thankless, necessary job.
8. This could be a super, preliminary training position for one to be considered as a possible candidate for the W.G.L.A. position. We'll have to think about that. [W.G.L.A. stands for the World's Greatest Living Authority, a pet name given to Gene's wife (Mary Ann) and one of our aunts, who "knew" all the answers to any question on a moment's notice.]

Several family members couldn't resist proposing ideas for the job title:

- Gary, Larry's oldest son: I propose the Hearing Efficacy Access Director—otherwise known as The HEAD.
- David, Larry's middle son: I'm so glad the interpreting fund is happening. And super big thanks to Wendy for coordinating. In the vein of Gary's suggestion, we could also call Wendy the BOSS, as in, the BMJ Office of Signer Scheduling.

So the Interpreter Fund was born, passed on to the next generation and thanks came in:

- Carolyn, Judy's sister-in-law: Thank you, Wendy, for handling this so efficiently for all of us. I appreciate having the interpreters so much! And thank you, everybody, for your contributions. Makes us deafies feel really accepted.

From time to time our BMJ families get emails similar to this one from Wendy:

Hey, all, it's that time of year again—time for your $30 annual contribution to the BMJ interpreter fund.... We've had a busy interpreting year, which means lots of family events! To date, our fund has paid for Passover, and I expect bills from both the wedding and Bar Mitzvah. I will send out an annual accounting of the total amount that has come in, and the total amount that has been paid out, and let you know of any funds still in the account (if any).... No, donations are not tax deductible, but they do contribute to open communication among all family members, which is truly priceless :)

Chapter Notes

Introduction

1. DEAF-WORLD is a compound ASL sign with no concise equivalent in written English. Traditionally authors have transcribed "...signs from signed languages with English glosses (approximate translation equivalents) in small capital letters. The dash in DEAF-WORLD indicates that this is a compound sign...." (Lane, Hoffmeister, Bahan, 1996, ix).

Chapter 5

1. In recent years, decades of sexual abuse in residential schools for the deaf have been reported in states throughout the country. Many of these accounts came from victims who are currently deaf adults. They stated they had spent many hours telling the adults, but it fell on "deaf ears" in spite of having been very detailed and graphic descriptions of the experiences. In addition, alumni of these schools also admitted the common practice of older students engaging in sex with younger ones. Deaf victims also knew they would be more likely to have to use the abusers as interpreters, if they chose to report the abuse, when the abuser was probably their only link to the hearing world.

Chapter 6

1. The name of the deaf school was changed to protect the identity of a specific location.

Chapter 7

1. To use the text relay service (TRS), deaf people use their TTYs to reach a third-party operator, a Communication Assistant (CA). The CA is the intermediary between the deaf person and the hearing person. The communication process would entail the following: the deaf person typed a message which the CA would read and speak to the hearing person. The same occurred in reverse: everything the hearing person spoke was typed to the deaf person and read on the TTY screen. The use of Go Ahead (GA) and Stop Keying (SK) are the key abbreviations used when the deaf person has finished typing and meant it was the hearing person's turn to respond. SK ended the conversation—the equivalent of hanging up. Video Relay Services (VRS) was an additional service using ASL interpreters rather than typists. Historically, TRS conversations were less desirable than the later VRS conversations for two main reasons: typing speeds are a great deal slower than spoken conversations, hampering a smooth give-and-take, and using typed English leads to many misunderstandings.

2. In July 2010, the 21st International Congress on the Education of the Deaf (ICED), hosted in Vancouver, British Columbia, formulated a Statement of Principle titled "A New Era: Deaf Participation and Collaboration," in which they stated their regrets to all the effects of the Milan Congress and pleaded for a global call to "accept and respect all languages and all

forms of communication" of deaf people (Milan 1880.com n.d.).

Chapter 9

1. Home signs are a gestural communication developed spontaneously in the home by deaf children who receive little or no input from a language model within their hearing families. As adults they continue to use home signs which do not share the traditional signs used by the conventional deaf community (Pinker 1994, 293).

2. In a spoken language, the sentence "I really like that dress on you" may have multiple meanings depending on the speaker's intent: sarcasm, enthusiasm, emphasis on the person rather than on someone else, emphasis on the dress rather than another item of clothing, etc. Vocal intonation, stress on a specific word, rising or lowering of pitch along with facial expression accomplish the speaker's goal. Visual-spatial languages like ASL show intent visually through facial expressions, intensity of signs including location and movement as well as specific non-manual mouth morphemes (merriam-webster.com/dictionary/monitor n.d.).

Chapter 10

1. A description of the BMJ Family Interpreter Fund is in Appendix D.

Chapter 12

1. RID's Code of Professional Conduct sets the minimal standards and guidelines for aspiring and certified interpreters to adhere to when interpreting in community settings, ensuring all parties are aware of the interpreting processes. Interpreting in family settings is generally at the discretion of the sibling-interpreter and the deaf sibling.

Bibliography

Abel, E. 2006. Mothers Raising Offspring According to Oralist Dictates. In Brueggemann, B., and Burch, S., eds. *Women and Deafness: Double Visions* (pp. 130–146). Washington, D.C.: Gallaudet University Press.

Atkins, D.V., ed. 1987. Families and Their Hearing-Impaired Children. *Volta Review* 89.

Bahan, B. 1989. It's Our World Too! In Wilcox, ed., *American Deaf Culture: An Anthology* (pp. 29–32). Burtonsville, MD: Linstok.

Bahan, B., Bauman, H., Montenegro, F., dirs. *Audism Unveiled*. 2008. (Motion picture).

Banta, E. 1979. The Families of Hearing Impaired Children: Siblings of Deaf-Blind Children. *Volta Review* 81, 363–369.

Bauman, H-Dirkson L., ed. 2008. *Open Your Eyes: Deaf Studies Talking*. Minneapolis: University of Minnesota Press.

_____. 2008. Postscript: Gallaudet Protests of 2006 and the Myths of In/ Exclusion. In H-Dirkson L. Bauman, *Open Your Eyes: Deaf Studies Talking* (pp. 327–336). Minneapolis: University of Minnesota Press.

Becker, G. 1980. *Growing Old in Silence*. Berkeley: University of California Press.

Berger, K. 2008. *The Developing Person Through the Life Span*. New York: Worth.

Beyond Silence Part I. Retrieved from Youtube.com: http://www.youtube.com/watch?v=18Qj93pfwXI.

Bienvenu, M. 1998. *Resistance to American Deaf Culture*, vol. 6. Retrieved from Deaf L—e-mail list server.

Binkard, B.A. 1987. *Brothers & Sisters Talk with PACER*. Minneapolis, MN: PACER Center.

Biopower. 2012. Retrieved June 15, 2013, from Wikipedia: http://en.wikipedia.org/wiki/Biopower#Foucault_and_the_concept_of_biopower.

Board, Mission Statement. n.d. Retrieved from Facundo Element: http://www.facundoelement.com/projecthumanity/board.php.

Brodsky, I.T., dir. 2007. *Hear and Now* (Motion picture).

Brueggemann, B.J. 2009. *Deaf Subjects: Between Identities and Places*. New York: New York University Press.

Cicirelli, V.G. 1995. *Sibling Relationships Across the Life Span*. New York: Plenum.

Code of Professional Conduct. n.d. Retrieved from Registry of Interpreters for the Deaf, http://rid.org/content/index.cfm/AID/66.

Collins, P.H. 2000. *Black Feminist Thought: Knowledge, Consciousness, and the Politics of Empowerment*. 2nd ed. New York: Routledge.

Congressional Hearing on Deaf Higher Education and Employment. 2013. Retrieved June 17, 2013, from Gallaudet.edu: http://www.gallaudet.edu/help_committee.xml.

Cued Speech Definition. n.d. Retrieved from National Cued Speech Association: http://www.cuedspeech.org/cued-speech-definition.

Cummins, J. 1991. Interdependence of First-and Second-Language Proficiency in Bilingual Children. In E. Bialystok, ed., *Language Processing in Bilingual Children* (pp. 70–89). Cambridge, UK: Cambridge University Press.

Danek, M. 1988. Deafness and Family Impact. In A. Del Orto, M. Gibsons, and P.D. Power, eds. *Family Interventions Throughout Chronic Illness and Disability* (pp. 120–135). New York: Springer.

Deafness Research Foundation News. 2012. The Race to Cure Hearing Loss in a Decade. *Hearing Health* 28, no. 1, pp. 38–39.

Drolsbaugh, M. 1997. *Deaf Again.* North Wales, PA: Handwave.

Durr, P. 2013. *PEOPLE OF THE EYE -... first, last, and all the time"—g. veditz 1910.* Retrieved July 10, 2013, from hand eyes.wordpress.com: https://handeyes.wordpress.com/tag/bermuda-triangle-of-oralism/.

Evans, J.F. 1995. Conversation at Home: A Case Study of a Young Deaf Child's Communication Experiences in a Family in Which All Others Can Hear. *American Annals of the Deaf* 140, no. 4, 324–332.

Featherstone, H. 1980. *A Difference in the Family: Life with a Disabled Child.* New York: Basic Books.

Feiges, L., and Weiss, M.J. 2004. *Sibling Stories: Reflections on Life with a Brother or Sister on the Autism Spectrum.* Shawnee Mission, KS: Autism Asperger Publishing.

Fillery, G. 2000. Deafness between Siblings; Barrier or Bond? *Deaf Worlds* 16, no. 1, 2–16.

_____. 2000. Deafness between Siblings; Barrier or Bond? Part Two: Case Studies. *Deaf Worlds* 16, no. 2, 39–48.

Foster, S. 1989. Social Alienation and Peer Identification: A Study of the Social Construction of Deafness. *Human Organization: Journal of the Society for Applied Anthropology* 48, no. 3, 226–235.

Foucault, M. 1994. *Power: The Essential Works of Michael Foucault, 1954–1984.* J.D. Faubion, ed. New York: New Press.

Frankenburg, F.R., Sloman, L. and Perry, A. 1985. Issues in the Therapy of Hearing Children with Deaf Parents: 3rd Annual Meeting of the Ontario Psychiatric Association (1982). *Canadian Journal of Psychiatry* 30, no. 2, 98–102.

Gaines, R., and Halpern-Felsher, B. 1995. Language Preference and Communication Development of a Hearing and Deaf Twin Pair. *American Annals of the Deaf* 140, no. 1, 477–555.

Gannon, J. 2002. *The Week The World Heard Gallaudet.* Washington, D.C.: Gallaudet University Press.

Garey, D., and Hott, L., dirs. 2007. *Deaf Jam* (Motion picture).

_____, dirs. 2007. *Through Deaf Eyes.* PBS DVD (Motion picture).

Gertz, G. 2008. Dysconscious Audism: A Theoretical Proposition. In H.-D.L. Bauman, *Open Your Eyes: Deaf Studies Talking* (pp. 219–234). Minneapolis: University of Minnesota Press.

Gold, D.T. 1989. Sibling Relationships: A Topology. *International Journal of Aging and Human Development* 28, 37–51.

Government Accountability Office (GAO). 2011. *May 2011 Report of Deaf and Hard of Hearing Children: Federal Support for Developing Language and Literacy.* Washington, D.C.: U.S. Government Printing Office.

Groce, N., and Whiting, J. 1985. *Everyone Here Spoke Sign Language: Hereditary Deafness on Martha's Vineyard.* Cambridge, MA: Harvard University Press.

Grosjean, F. 1982. *Life with Two Languages.* Cambridge: Harvard University Press.

Guilbeau, N. 2012. *Siblings Site: The Birth Order Theory.* Retrieved from BellaOnLine: the Voice of Women: http://www.bellaonline.com/articles/art22888.asp.

Gustason, G. 1990. Signing Exact English. In H. Bornstein, Ed., *Manual Communication: Implications for Education* (pp. 108–127). Washington, D.C.: Gallaudet University Press.

Hall, W., and Andrews, S. 1989. At Home with Mothers of Young Children with Hearing Impairment in Jamaica; A Case Study. *Topics in Early Childhood Special Education* 9, no. 3, 128–134.

Higgins, P. 1980. *Outsiders in a Hearing World: A Sociology of Deafness.* Newbury Park, CA: SAGE.

Holcomb, T.K., and Mindless, A. 2009. *See*

What I Mean: Differences between Deaf and Hearing Cultures (motion picture). Treehouse Video, LLC.

_____. 2013. *Introduction to American Deaf Culture.* New York: Oxford University Press.

Humphries, T. 1977. *Communicating Across Cultures (deaf-/hearing) and Language Learning.* PhD dissertation, Union Institute and University, Cincinnati, OH.

_____, and Humphies, J. 2011. Deaf in the Time of the Cochlea. *Journal of Deaf Studies and Deaf Education, Special Section on Deaf Studies* 16, no. 2, 153–164.

ICED 2010 Statement. n.d. Retrieved April 18, 2013, from milan1880.com: www.milan1880.com/iced2010statement.html.

Israelite, N.K. 1985. Sibling Reaction to a Hearing Impaired Child in the Family. *Journal of Rehabilitation of the Deaf* 18, no. 3, 1–5.

_____. 1986. Hearing-Impaired Children and the Psychological Functioning of Their Normal-Hearing Siblings. *Volta Review* 88, 47–54.

It's My Life. Family, Birth Order: What Is "Birth Order"? (n.d.). Retrieved from pbskids.org: http://pbskids.org/itsmylife/family/birthorder/index.html.

Jennison, L. 1997. Brotherly Bonds, Lifetime Friends: William, Mark, Kevin and Patrick Jennison. *The Endeavor* 1 (winter).

Judy Doesn't Want to Go to School: The Family and School Attendance. October 1986. *Exceptional Parent* 16, no. 6, 47–52.

Kennedy, H. 1985. Growing Up with a Handicapped Sibling. Presented at the Meeting of the Association for Child Psychoanalysis, Chicago, March 1984. *The Psychoanalytic Study of the Child* 40, 255–274.

Keydel, C. 1988. The Impact of a Handicapped Child on Adolescent Siblings: Implications for Professional Intervention. In A. Dell Orto, M. Gibbons and P. Power, eds. *Family Interventions Throughout Chronic Illness and Disability* (pp. 201–215). New York: Springer.

Klein, S.D., and Schleifer, M.J., eds. 1993. *It Isn't Fair! Siblings of Children with Disabilities.* Westport, Connecticut: Exceptional Parent Press.

Kluger, J. 2006. The New Science of Siblings. *TIME* (July 10): pp. 47–55.

_____. 2011. *The Sibling Effect: What the Bonds Among Brothers and Sisters Reveal About Us.* . New York: Riverhead.

Konig, T.J. 1986. A Special Brother. *Sibling Information Network Newsletter* 5, no. 1, 4.

Kretschmer, R.R., and Kretschmer, L.W. 1979. The Acquisition of Linguistic and Communicative Competence: Parent-Child Interactions. *Volta Review* 81, 306–322.

Ladd, P. 2003. *Understanding Deaf Culture: In Search of Deafhood.* Clevedon, UK: Multilingual Matters.

Lalou, S. (producer), N. Philibert (writer and director). 1994. *Le pays des sourds (In the Land of the Deaf).* New York: Kino International. VHS (Motion picture).

Lane, H., Hoffmeister, R., and Bahan, B. 1996. *A Journey into the Deaf-World.* San Diego: DawnSign Press.

_____. 1999. *The Mask of Benevolence: Disabling the Deaf Community.* San Diego: DawnSign Press.

Leigh, I., and Christiansen, J. 2002. *Cochlear Implants in Children: Ethics and Choices.* Washington, D.C.: Gallaudet University Press.

_____, 2009. *A Lens on Deaf Identities: Perspectives on Deafness.* New York: Oxford University Press.

Leviticus 19:23. Bible n.d.

Luetke-Stahlman, H. B. 1992. Yes, Siblings Can Help. *Perspectives in Education and Deafness* 10, no. 5, 9–11.

Luterman, D.M. 1987. *Deafness in the Family.* Austin: Pro-ed.

_____, and Ross, M. 1991. *When Your Child Is Deaf: A Guide for Parents.* Parkton, MD: York.

McQuillan, L.A., and Atherton, M. 2007. Sibling Relationships in a Mixed Deaf/hearing Family. *Deaf World* 22, 71–85.

Mahshie, S. 1997. *A First Language: Whose Choice Is It?* Retrieved from Laurent Clerc National Deaf Education Center, Gallaudet University, Washington, D.C.:

http://www.tep.ucsd.edu/about/Cours es/EDS342A/SI-AFirstLanguage.pdf

Malcolm, R.L. 1990. My Sister is Deaf, and What About Me? Meeting the Needs of Siblings. *Perspectives in Education and Deafness* 9, no. 1, 12–14.

Marschark, M. 1997. *Raising and Educating a Deaf Child.* New York: Oxford University Press.

_____, and Hauser, P. 2012. *What Parents and Teachers Need to Know: How Deaf Children Learn.* New York: Oxford University Press.

Meadow-Orlans, K.P., Mertens, D.M., and Sass-Lehrer, M.A. 2002. *Parents and Their Deaf Children: The Early Years.* Washington, D.C.: Gallaudet University Press.

Merriam-Webster Online Dictionary. (n.d.) Monitor. Retrieved from http://www.m erriam-webster.com/dictionary/monitor.

Meyer, D.J., Vadasy, P.F., and Fewell, R.R. 1985. *Living with a Brother or Sister with Special Needs: A Book for Sibs.* Baltimore: Woodbine House.

_____. 1996. *Living with a Brother or Sister with Special Needs: A Book for Sibs.* 2nd ed., revised and expanded. Seattle: University of Washington Press.

_____. 1998. Sibling Support Project. Retrieved from http://www.siblingsuppo rt.org/.

Miller, S. 1985. Siblings. *Sibling Information Network Newsletter* 4, no. 3, 4.

Modern Language Association Press Release. December 8, 2010. *Modern Language Association.* Retrieved June 18, 2013, from Enrollments in Languages Other Than English in United States Institutions of Higher Education, Fall 2009: http://www.mla.org/pdf/2009_ enrollment_survey_pr.pdf.

Mow, S. 1989. How Do You Dance Without Music? In S. Wilcox, ed., *American Deaf Culture: An Anthology* (pp. 33–44). Burtonsville, MD: Linstok.

Murphy, A.T. 1979. The Families of Handicapped Children: Context for Disability. *Volta Review* 81, 265–277.

_____. 1979. Members of the Family: Sisters and Brothers of Handicapped Children. *Volta Review* 81, 352–362.

National Organization of the Deaf. (n.d.) About Us. Retrieved from https://www. nad.org/about-us.

Office of Communications, Gallaudet University. 2013. *Gallaudet Today Magazine* (Spring).

Oliva, G. 2004. *Alone in the Mainstream: A Deaf Woman Remembers Public School.* Washington, D.C.: Gallaudet University Press.

One Hundred Seventh Congress of the United States of America. *No Child Left Behind Act of 2001.* Retrieved June 14, 2013, from Department of Education: http://www2.ed.gov/policy/elsec/leg/e sea02/beginning.html#sec1.

Padden, C., and Humphries, T. 1988. *Deaf in America: Voices from a Culture.* Cambridge: Harvard University Press.

_____. 1989. The Deaf Community and the Culture of Deaf People. In S. Wilcox, *American Deaf Culture: An Anthology* (pp. 1–16). Burtonsville, MD: Linstok.

_____. 2005. *Inside Deaf Culture.* Cambridge: Harvard University Press.

Parnes, A. 2009. Update on ADARA Communication Access Task Force. *Adara Update: Professionals Networking for Excellence in Service Delivery with Individuals who are Deaf or hard of Hearing.*

Pinker, S. 1994. *The Language Instinct: How the Mind Creates Language.* New York: W. Morrow.

Pizzo, R. 2001. *Growing Up Deaf: Issues of Communication in a Hearing World.* Philadelphia: Xlibris.

Pollard, R. 1993–94. Cross Cultural Ethics in the Conduct of Deafness Research. *Journal of the American Deafness and Rehabilitation Association* 27, no. 3, 29–38.

Powell, T. 1993, and Gallagher, P. 1993. *Brothers and Sisters—A Special Part of Exceptional Families,* 2nd ed. Baltimore: Paul H. Brookes.

Preston, P. 1994. *Mother Father Deaf: Living Between Sound and Silence.* Cambridge: Harvard University Press.

Pro-Tactile: The Deaf-Blind Way. Retrieved from http:www.protactile.org.

Ritchie, D.A. 1995. *Doing Oral History.* New York: Twayne.

Robbins, C. 2002. Solo Dining While Growing Up. In T. Stremlau, ed., *The Deaf Way II Anthology: A Literary Collection by Deaf and Hard of Hearing Writers* (p. 6). Washington, D.C.: Gallaudet University Press.

Robinson, M.J. 1979. Sink or Swim: The Single-Parent Family with a Deaf Child. *Volta Review* 81, 370–377.

Rodman, J. 2011. Why Aren't They Watching Me? *RID VIEWS* 28, no. 3, 36–37.

Rodriguez, M.S., and Lana, E.T. 1996. Children and Their Communication Partners. *American Annals of the Deaf* 141, no. 3, 245–251.

Roffe, H. 2007. Life With Hearing Loss. *Hearing Health* (Spring): 35–37.

Sacks, O. 1989. *Seeing Voices: A Journey into the World of the Deaf.* Berkeley: University of California Press.

Schein, J., M. Delk, H. Lipman, F. Bowe, and T. Freebairn. 1976. *Continuing Education of Deaf Adults: Report of a Survey Conducted for Bureau of Education for the Handicapped United States Office of Education.* New York University School of Education, Deafness Research & Training Center.

Schlesinger, H.S., and Meadow, K.P. 1972. *Sound and Sign: Childhood Deafness and Mental Health.* Berkeley: University of California Press.

Schwirian, P. 1976. Effects of the Presence of a Hearing-Impaired Preschool Child in the Family on Behavior Patterns of Older "Normal" Siblings. *American Annals of the Deaf* 121, no. 4, 373–380.

See the Sound. n.d. Retrieved from http://seethesound.org.

Seiberlich, A. 2004. *WITNESSING OPPRESSION. Respect in the Face of Witnessing Oppression: It Can Be Done.* Retrieved from Leadership Institute: www.leadershipinstitute.biz/articles.html.

Seligman, M., and Darling, R. *Ordinary Families, Special Children: A Systems Approach to Childhood Disability*, 2nd ed. New York: Guilford.

Shapiro, B. 1983. Informational Interviews. *Sibling Information Network Newsletter* 2, no. 1, p. 5.

Sheridan, M. A. 2001. *Inner Lives of Deaf Children: Interviews and Analysis.* Washington, D.C.: Gallaudet University Press.

_____. 2008. *Deaf Adolescents: Inner Lives and Lifeworld Development.* Washington, D.C.: Gallaudet University Press.

Sibling Interviews. 1982. Videotape. Produced by New Jersey Parents fo Deaf Awareness.

Siblings Who Cope with Special Brothers and Sisters. 1997. *The Endeavor*, p. 1.

Silver, A. 1997. *Thou Shalt Speak For, With, By, and Of.* A Deaf American Monograph 47, National Association of the Deaf, 53–57.

Singleton, J.L., and Morgan, D.D. 2006. Natural Signed Language Acquisition Within the Social Context of the Classroom. In B. Schick, M. Marschark, and P. Spencer, eds. *Advances in the Sign Language Development of Deaf Children* (pp. 344–375). New York: Oxford University Press.

Slesser, S. 1994. Deaf Adults with Hearing Siblings—Communication and Attitudes. *Deafness* 3, no. 10, 6–10.

Smith, R.C. 1996. *A Case About Amy.* Philadelphia: Temple University Press.

Solomon, A. 2012. *Far from the Tree.* New York: Scribner.

Spencer, P.E., C.J. Erting, and M. Marschark. 2000. *The Deaf Child in the Family and at School: Essays in Honor of Kathryn P. Meadow-Orlans.* Mahway, NJ: Lawrence Erlbaum Associates.

Strol, M.G. 2011. *MLK and the Disability Rights Movement.* Retrieved October 16, 2013, from Disability Rights Galaxy: http://www.disabilityrightsgalaxy.com/mlk-and-the-disability-rights-movement.

Tapper, J., and Sandell, C. 2006. *Is Deaf University President Not 'Deaf Enough?'* Retrieved May 10, 2013, from ABC News: http://abcnews.go.com/WNT/story?id=1947073&page=1.

Tattersall, H.Y. 2003. Exploring the impact on hearing children of having a deaf sibling. *Deafness and Education International* 5, no. 2, 108–122.

Tolle, E. 2005. *A New Earth: Awakening to Your Life's Purpose.* New York: Penguin.

Tribute to Marie Jean Philip. n.d. Retrieved June 13, 2013, from The Learning Center for the Deaf: http://www.tlcdeaf. org/page.cfm?p=501.

Tuccoli, T. 2008. *Hearing Privilege at Gallaudet?* Master's thesis, Gallaudet University, Washington, D.C.

Valli, C., and Lucas C. 1995. *Linguistics of American Sign Language.* 2nd ed. Washington, D.C.: Gallaudet University Press.

Verghese, A. 2009. *Cutting for Stone.* New York: Vintage Books.

Videophone. n.d. Retrieved June 6, 2013, from Wikipedia: http://en.wikipedia.o rg/wiki/Videophone.

White, S.J. 1984. *Antecedents of Language Functioning in the Deaf: Implications for Early Intervention.* Project Summary (ERIC Report ED 243–297 EC 162–425), Lexington School for the Deaf, New York.

Wiesel, E. 1986. One Must Not Forget. *US News & World Reports* (October 27), p. 68.

Wilcox, S. 1989. *American Deaf Culture: An Anthology.* Burtonsville, MD: Linstok.

Williams, L. 1988. College for Deaf Is Shut by Protest Over President, Special to the *New York Times*, March 8. Retrieved from NYTimes.com: http://www.nyti mes.com/1988/03/08/us/college-for-d eaf-is-shut-by-protest-over-president. html?src=pm.

Wrigley, O. 1996. *The Politics of Deafness.* Washington, D.C.: Gallaudet University Press.

Index